THE CONTROL OF GROWTH AND FORM:

A Study of the Epidermal Cell in an Insect

The Control of Growth and Form:

A STUDY OF THE EPIDERMAL CELL IN AN INSECT

✦✦✦✦✦✦✦✦✦✦✦✦✦✦✦✦✦

By V. B. Wigglesworth

M.D., F.R.S.

Quick Professor of Biology in the University of Cambridge and *Director of the Agricultural Research Council Unit of Insect Physiology*

Cornell University Press

ITHACA, NEW YORK

PRINTED IN THE UNITED STATES OF AMERICA
BY CAYUGA PRESS, INC.

Preface

THE title of this small book can scarcely fail to call to mind that great work of D'Arcy Wentworth Thompson *On Growth and Form,* which ran to 1116 pages in its second edition. In that book D'Arcy Thompson sought to discuss the many ways in which physical and mathematical laws control or influence the form of growing animals. The six brief essays that are here presented have a more modest aim. They rest on the assumption that the physiological control of growth and form is based on principles that are common to all animals. The epidermal cell in an insect has been chosen as the text around which these principles can be displayed and as the medium in which their workings can be studied. Such a limitation has obvious shortcomings. It has the merit of confining the argument within manageable bounds and thus permitting within a small compass the consideration of both facts and theory.

Many of the facts and ideas that are discussed were included in an earlier monograph, *The Physiology of Insect Metamorphosis.* But these general conceptions have now been sifted from the extensive literature on metamorphosis and developed as a self-contained thesis on growth and form.

The argument as here presented is based on six Messenger

Lectures "directed to a general audience" which I was invited to give at Cornell University in the fall of 1958. I should like to take this opportunity of expressing my strong sense of the high distinction conferred by such an invitation and my warm appreciation of all the kindness I enjoyed during my visit to Cornell.

V. B. W.

University of Cambridge
May 1959

Contents

Preface v
I The Epidermal Cell 1
II The Capacity for Differentiation 21
III Hormones and the Control of Growth 43
IV Hormones and the Control of Form 67
V Polymorphism 91
VI The Integration of Growth 105
References 125
Index 139

THE CONTROL OF GROWTH AND FORM:

A Study of the Epidermal Cell in an Insect

1 · The Epidermal Cell

ANY satisfactory account of growth should cover all its manifestations in plants and animals.

We should deal first with the viruses, which seem to have separated out a single function of the living organism, nucleic acid replication and protein synthesis, and concentrated on the perfection of that, relying for everything else upon the living system of their host.

Then we should discuss the growth of bacteria, which are infinitely more complex, with an individuality of a higher order and with systems of heredity approximating to those of higher animals and plants. We should find that a large part of the life and growth of bacteria can be described in terms of enzyme synthesis and adaptation.

With the protozoa we reach much greater heights of complexity. Although unicellular, they have a genetic system, the study of which, in *Paramoecium*, for example, has thrown light on the relative importance of nuclear genes and cytoplasmic factors in the inheritance of characters. Although containing but a single nucleus (or, rather, a macro- and a micronucleus), the protozoa exhibit structures of the most diverse kinds which vie in complexity with those of multicellular

animals and which pose the same problems of form production or morphogenesis.

In amoebae we find the form of the body being influenced
by both nucleus and cytoplasm. By transferring the isolated
nucleus of one species of amoeba to the isolated cytoplasm of
another species, it has been shown that many of the characters
of the resulting "hybrid" or chimaera are determined by the
cytoplasm, and relatively few by the nucleus.[18]

For such experimental studies of morphogenesis the unicellular alga *Acetabularia* has provided wonderful material.
The single nucleus at the base of the stolon is responsible for
the specific form of the "umbrella" at the apex: if the nucleus
of one species is replaced by that of another, the form of the
"umbrella" becomes that appropriate to the new nucleus. But
the original nuclear influence can persist for some little time in
the cytoplasm, for an isolated segment of stolon will still form
a small umbrella of the normal specific character.

When we come to multicellular organisms, the same problems reappear—problems of polarity and of gradients in morphogenetic potential. There is, for example, an extensive
literature that deals with regeneration in planarians, notably
with the factors which ensure that, after extirpation of fragments of the body, a new head is developed only at the front
end. Even if a little window is cut in the body of the worm,
it is the posterior margin of this window, which is now the
leading edge of a certain region of the body, that develops a
second small head. How does a head in continuity with the
rest of the body prevent the appearance of a new head? And
why do two heads form if the decapitated worm is split lengthways?

So we are led on to the general problems of the co-ordination of cells and their specialization or differentiation to

perform different functions. We have the slime mould *Acrasia* which can exist in the form of free and independent amoeboid cells living a life of their own. Then, under the influence of a specific chemical substance, they will converge to one focus, associate together, and jointly build an erect process of constant form which will develop into a fruiting body or sporangium.

We find a somewhat similar phenomenon in the sponges, where the organism can be dissociated into its individual cells, and these forced through a fine filter, after which process they will reassociate with one another and build a new sponge.

But it is the development of embryos which has provided most of the material for the experimental study of growth or developmental physiology. There is a vast literature on the differentiation of the segmenting egg cell in echinoderms, on the factors which determine the formation of the animal and vegetable poles of the embryo, and on the related problem of the role of the different regions of the cytoplasm in controlling the future fate of the various cell lines which receive these special cytoplasmic parts.

In the embryos of amphibia and other vertebrates there is the phenomenon of induction: the effect of apparent chemical substances coming from the roof of the archenteron in provoking the appearance of a nerve cord rudiment in the embryo. This problem and the further problems of "induction" in later development have a vast literature dating from the time of Roux and of Spemann.

Although there are some who regard the science of genetics as the esoteric preserve of those engaged in the study of Mendelian ratios and who almost deny the relevance of physiology, my sympathies are with Richard Goldschmidt who has so often emphasized that genetics is really just a part of the general problem of growth. To find out how genes bring about their effects, in deciding what characters shall appear as growth proceeds, is one of the most informative methods of discovering something about the nature of the growth process itself.

In addition, growth involves maintenance and repair. At its simplest, this means the healing of wounds; in its more extreme manifestations, the regeneration of extirpated appendages. In many arthropods, if an antenna or a leg is removed, a new antenna or a new leg is formed. But why, when an antenna is removed, does the insect sometimes regenerate a leg?

In some animals the form of the body is strikingly influenced by disturbances in hormone secretion; and thus the whole field of hormones and morphogenesis falls within our theme. Hormones, as well-recognized products of endocrine glands, merge into diffusible chemical factors which still await proper characterization. Among animals we see the most striking metamorphoses brought about by simple changes in hormone secretion. In plants we see the closely similar phenomenon of flowering, the control of which is still little understood.

Normal growth is possible only because growth is restrained: cells multiply up to a point and then stop. But something may go wrong with this restraint. Cells, instead of halting when they meet neighbouring cells and settling down in harmony, continue to multiply and migrate until the normal cells are swamped and overcome. That is the problem of tumour formation and malignant growth, the full understanding of which must wait upon an understanding of all these other types of controlled growth upon which we have been reflecting.

It is evident enough that the study of growth embraces a vast section of biology. Any attempt to cover this whole field in six brief essays could give only a superficial review of a few facts which at no point would come anywhere near the heart of the problem. But one thing is certain: if we really understood a single one of these growth phenomena, we should have made a very long step toward understanding all. The only way in which we can hope to penetrate at all deeply into the subject is to take a limited part of it and consider that in some detail.

Most of the basic phenomena of life are summed up in the amoeba—sometimes referred to as a "simple animal." But the amoeba is an almost impossibly difficult animal to use in the study of physiology, for all the physiological functions are concentrated in a single cell, a cell of baffling complexity. The deepest insight into the working of cells has been obtained in those that are most specialized—nerve axons, muscle fibres, and the like, which have become modified to perform a single function.

In other words, there is much to be said for starting with the specialized parts of a complex animal, rather than with an animal which has all the functions but none of the differentiated structures. It is on these grounds that I would hope to justify myself in entitling this book "The Control of Growth and Form" and yet writing only about the insect.

But my survey is not going to be as broad as that. There must be some two million or more sorts of insects in the world, and they extend over a greater range of size and of form than any other group of animals. We must restrict ourselves to something more manageable. I propose to deal mainly with a single insect, *Rhodnius prolixus*. This is a member of the Triatomidae, close relatives of the Reduviidae of the order Hemiptera, the bugs. It is a blood-sucking insect, a native of Venezuela, where it is responsible for carrying Chagas's disease, a serious form of trypanosomiasis in human beings. After hatching from the egg, *Rhodnius* goes through five larval stages before it becomes adult. The fourth larval stage, the fifth larval stage, measuring about 13 mm. in length, and the adult *Rhodnius,* about 2 cm. long, are illustrated in Plate I.

Insects have an exceedingly complex structure, with elaborate internal organs: a circulatory and a respiratory system; a digestive system with a whole range of enzymes; an excretory system; and sense organs of incredible complexity, linked by way of a highly evolved nervous system to muscles immensely more numerous and complex than those in the human body, for example. The whole mechanism is operated through systems of enzymes which closely resemble those described in vertebrate animals. We cannot cope with such complexity in six chapters.

The outward form of the insect is fixed by the form of its external skeleton or cuticle. This cuticle is the product of a single layer of epidermal cells. Thus in the ultimate analysis it is the functional activity of the epidermal cell which is mainly responsible for the growth and form of the insect. The control of growth resolves itself into the control of the enzyme system contained within this cell. In the resting state the epidermal cell is a thin and flattened attenuated object, the nucleus containing a small nucleolus, the cytoplasm with some scattered granular and filamentous mitochondria and a little ribonucleic acid (Fig. 1; Plate II, *a*). But it is a cell with great potentialities, for which I have come to entertain a profound respect.

I must first endeavour to convey some idea of what this cell does, in co-operation with its neighbours, during each cycle of growth. For growth in the insect takes place in cycles: the cuticle can be stretched to some extent, but it cannot grow. For

[6]

Plate I

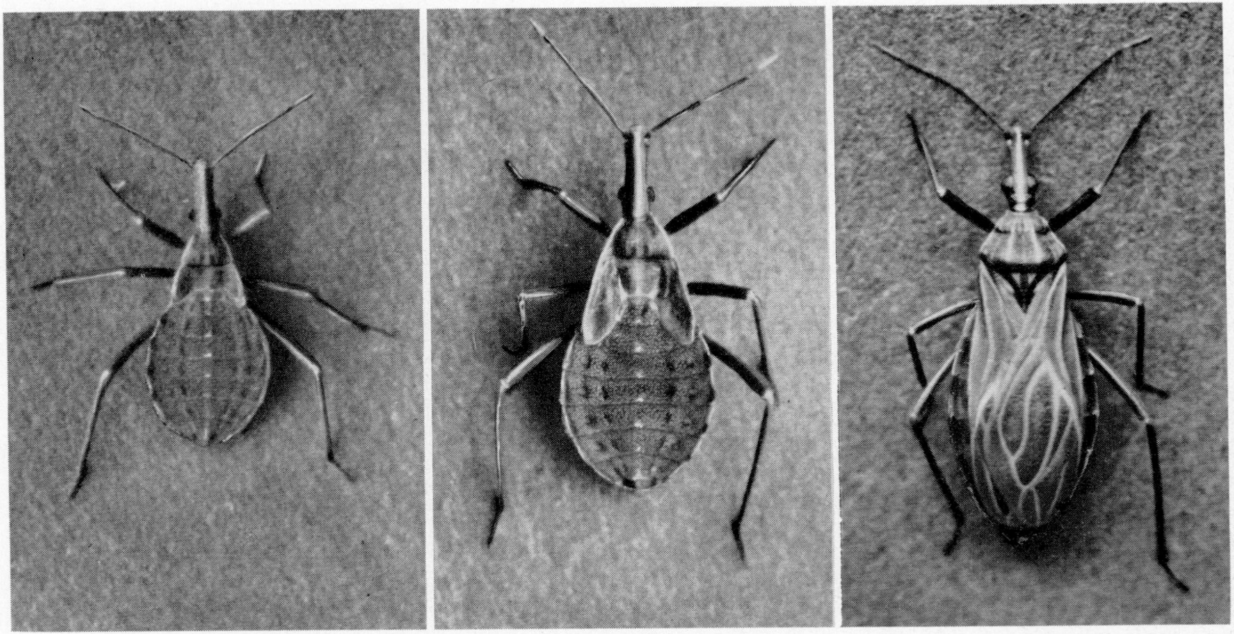

a, 4th-stage larva of *Rhodnius*.　　　b, 5th-stage larva.　　　c, adult *Rhodnius*.

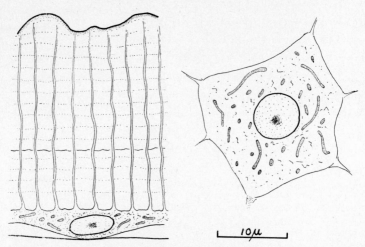

Fig. 1. The resting epidermal cell in *Rhodnius* larva. Transverse section, to the left, shows the basement membrame below the cell and the pore canals running vertically through the cuticle. Horizontal view, to the right, shows the nucleus with small nucleolus and granular and filamentous mitochondria in the cytoplasm.

true growth to occur it must therefore be cast off and a new and larger cuticle formed below. It is this process, the moulting cycle, which must first be described.

Rhodnius is a convenient insect for observations of this kind because it takes only a single meal of blood in each moulting cycle. It ingests a meal which may amount to twelve times its own weight,[14] and that supplies all the material it needs to lay down its enlarged cuticle and to provide for the corresponding growth of all its internal parts. And when this process is complete, the insect usually carries over sufficient reserves to maintain it (in the absence of further growth) for another five or six months.

As we shall see later, growth begins within a few hours after a fresh meal has been taken. The epidermal cells, which

[8]

are exceedingly attenuated in the starving insect, enlarge until they become cubical or columnar and they add a little more substance to the inner layers of the existing cuticle (Fig. 2).[120] Then, about six or seven days after feeding, they are found to have multiplied considerably and to have detached themselves from the old cuticle. By eight or nine days after feeding, the epidermal cells begin to lay down the new cuticle.

This is an exceedingly complex process which is far from being adequately understood. First, a refractile layer of something less than 1μ thick is deposited on the surface of the cell. This layer, the "cuticulin" layer, which is composed of lipoprotein, expands by some unknown mechanism so that it is thrown into folds.[83] The inner layers are then secreted. These are composed of protein and chitin, closely associated together, perhaps chemically bound.[30] Both protein and chitin are in the form of elongated crystallites, disposed at random in superimposed laminae. As a result of this arrangement these layers are birefringent when viewed tangentially.

From the cells there arise cytoplasmic processes which extend almost to the surface. The chitin and protein of the cuticle are laid down around these processes which come to form slender canals, the so-called pore canals, that run a more or less convoluted course through the cuticle—just as bone or dentine are traversed by the Haversian or dentine canals. Some fifty to sixty of these filaments spring from a single cell.[83, 93]

The deposition of chitin and protein continues for five or six days. Then the epidermal cells take on a new function. The space between the old cuticle and the new is occupied by a thin film of fluid. This fluid now comes to contain a proteolytic and a chitinolytic enzyme, secreted by the epidermal cells through the new cuticle, perhaps by way of the pore canals. These enzymes digest the inner layers of the old cuticle. If a

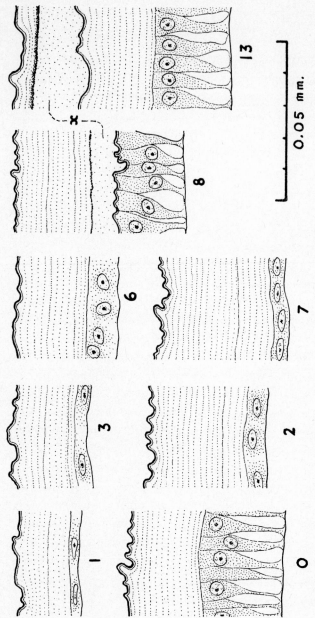

Fig. 2. Transverse sections through the integument of 4th-stage and 5th-stage larvae of *Rhodnius* at different periods in the moulting cycle. 1, one day after feeding; 3, 6, 8, 13, three, six, eight, and thirteen days after feeding. 0, 5th-stage larva on day of moulting (fourteen days after feeding); 2, 7, two days and seven days after moulting. *x* indicates the moulting fluid between the old and the new cuticles.

0.05 mm.

fragment of protein stained with congo red is inserted into this space, it is digested and the dye diffuses out.[83] Digestion proceeds until only the thin outermost parts of the old cuticle remain; more than 90 per cent of the cuticle may be dissolved. The products of digestion are absorbed through the new cuticle into the body of the insect and presumably utilized again in cuticle formation or for energy production. In other insects a chitinase and protease have been demonstrated in the extracted moulting fluid.[51]

Before the undigested residue of the old cuticle is shed, further changes take place in the new cuticle. The outer parts that are to become hard and horny are heavily impregnated with protein. This protein is associated with phenolic substances with two or more phenolic groups. There is still some doubt whether these di- or polyphenols are an integral part of the protein of the cuticle or whether they are free and soluble materials. It seems more likely that they are built into the protein.[10, 108]

Similar proteinaceous material rich in phenolic groups is discharged from the ends of the pore canals and spreads out to form a viscid layer over the surface. This layer, sometimes called the "polyphenol layer," like the phenolic materials in the cuticle, is readily demonstrated by its intensely reducing properties towards ammoniacal silver hydroxide.[93, 95]

Finally, a layer of crystalline wax forms over the surface of the silver-reducing layer. These waxes are likewise a product of the epidermal cells and are secreted through the newly formed cuticle. They have the all-important property of waterproofing the insect,[4, 5, 91] and it is obviously essential that this waterproofing process should be complete before the old skin is shed and the new cuticle exposed to the air.

The critical moment has now arrived. The insect is ready

to moult the remains of its old skin. The muscles are detached from their old insertions into the cuticle, and the distal processes of the sense cells rupture and lose their connection with the innervated hairs of the old cuticle.[101] The insect expands its new cuticle by swallowing large amounts of air and then, contracting its abdomen so as to press the body fluids forward into the thorax, it splits the fragile remains of its old skin and draws itself out.

The new cuticle is still soft and colourless; and while it is in this state, the insect swallows more air and, by hydrostatic pressure as before, it proceeds to expand its appendages to their full size and shape. If it is the adult insect that is being produced, the crumpled wings are unfolded and expanded by this same internal pressure to form membranous sheets.

As this process is going on, that is, during the first half hour after moulting, another layer is formed on the cuticle. Like the "cuticulin" layer, this also appears to be a lipoprotein material of some kind. It is poured out from numerous dermal glands whose ducts everywhere pierce the cuticle, and it spreads evenly over the surface to form a thin protective covering for the waterproofing wax. We commonly refer to this as the "cement" layer.[93]

Finally, within the next few hours, the cuticle becomes hardened and darkened. Tyrosinase, secreted by the epidermal cells, leads to melanin formation and blackening in the substance of the cuticle in certain regions. And in the outer parts of the cuticle, which are destined to become horny and amber coloured, the diphenols are oxidized to quinones. These react with the amino, imino, and sulphydryl groups of the protein chains, linking these chains together to form a hard plastic.[59]

The hydrophil reactive groups of the protein are thus blocked, and what was a soft, colourless, and soluble material becomes converted into a hard, insoluble, brown or amber coloured, and lipophil substance. This is the process of quinone tanning, well known in the manufacture of leather from hides. But in the insect, as Pryor, who first described this process, has said, the animal tans its own skin.

The resulting product has much in common with the hard keratin of hair or horn, but whereas in keratin the protein chains are linked together by sulphur bridges, in the hard substance of the cuticle, which is known as "sclerotin," the proteins are bound together through benzene rings.

Even at this stage the process is not yet complete, for only about one half to two thirds of the total thickness of the cuticle has been formed. The remaining part is laid down mainly during the next five or six days.

That is a highly simplified account of the process of cuticle formation in *Rhodnius*. The true nature of most of the chemical changes taking place is not known, and they are certainly more complex than I have indicated. But this brief summary will serve to emphasize the amazing range of activities of the epidermal cell, which is to be the hero of our plot (Fig. 3).

To recapitulate: this cell secretes the lipoprotein or cuticulin of the epicuticle; it then secretes the protein and chitin of the inner layers. It secretes and discharges the chitinase and pro-teinase which digest the inner layers of the old cuticle; and it reabsorbs the products of digestion. It produces the phenolic compounds which will later be responsible for hardening and darkening and then the long-chain waxes to waterproof the surface. Finally, it produces the phenol oxidase enzymes which lead to melanization and tanning. And all these processes are integrated and timed so that they follow one another in orderly sequence and synchronously in all parts of the body.

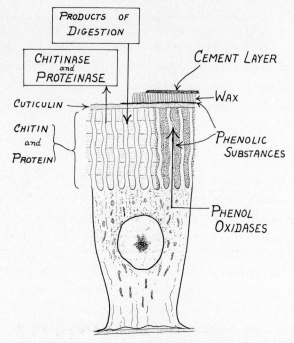

Fig. 3. Schematic figure of the epidermal cell, to summarize the structure and composition of the cuticle and the activities of the cell during the moulting cycle.

At this point it will be well to say a little about some of the neighbouring cells which co-operate with the ordinary epidermal cell in carrying out these functions (Fig. 4).

The epidermal cells rest upon a basement membrane. It may be that they contribute to its formation; but there seems little doubt that it is the haemocytes or blood cells which are mainly responsible. This membrane consists of a complex material containing protein, carbohydrate, and perhaps lipid. Just at the time when the epidermal cells have completed their multiplication and are about to begin to deposit the new

PLATE II

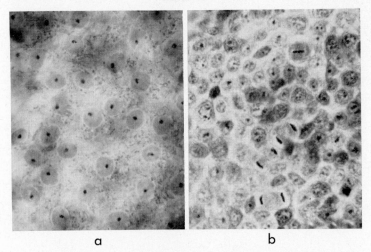

a   b

a, epidermal cells in the abdomen of *Rhodnius* 4th-stage larva in the resting state with small nucleoli and slender mitochondria. (Whole mount: osmium-ethyl gallate method of staining.)

b, the same at 5 days after feeding; mitosis in progress in the epidermis. (Whole mount: haematoxylin.)

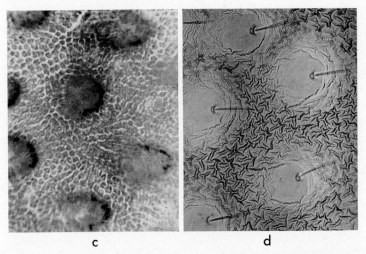

c   d

c, distribution of epidermal cells in 5th-stage larva of *Rhodnius* in relation to the plaques. (The plaques are convex; hence the cells below them are out of focus.)

d, surface view of abdominal cuticle in 5th-stage larva of *Rhodnius* showing plaques, bristles, and stellate folds in the epicuticle.

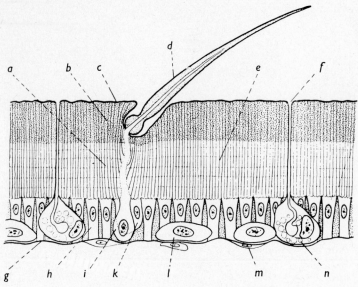

Fig. 4. Ideal section of the cuticle and the underlying cells. *a,* laminated endocuticle; *b,* exocuticle; *c,* epicuticle; *d,* bristle; *e,* pore canals; *f,* duct of dermal glands; *g,* basement membrane; *h,* epidermal cell; *i,* trichogen cell; *k,* tormogen cell; *l,* oenocyte; *m,* haemocyte adherent to basement membrane; *n,* dermal gland. The sense cell and axon of the bristle have been omitted.

cuticle, the haemocytes congregate in great numbers on the basement membrane and spread out in stellate form upon it (Fig. 5). These cells contain rounded or oval deposits of apparently the same chemical nature as the basement membrane (that is, they are osmiophil and PAS-positive and contain protein), and the cells can be seen to discharge these inclusions to add them to the substance of the membrane (Plate III, *a, b*).[106]

Between the epidermal cells and the basement membrane are some very large cells termed oenocytes (Plate III, *c, d*). These also go through a cycle of changes during moulting. [83, 93]

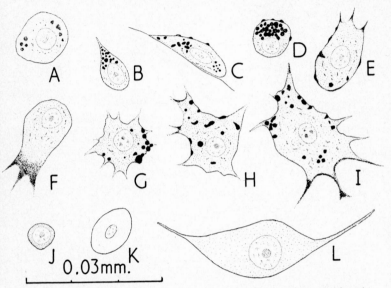

Fig. 5. Haemocytes below the basement membrane of the epidermis in 4th-stage larva of *Rhodnius* at 7 days after feeding. A-I, amoebocytes containing mucopolysaccharide inclusions stained with periodic acid—Schiff technique. The cells show various stages in the extrusion of the inclusions to form the basement mmbrane. J-L, other types of blood cells.

They enlarge rapidly in the early stages, reaching their greatest dimensions just before the lipoprotein epicuticle is laid down. At this time they may measure as much as 100μ in diameter. The staining properties of the oenocytes show that they also contain lipoprotein. They give out processes which appear to discharge this material among the epidermal cells. Then they diminish in size again (Fig. 6).

The conclusion drawn from these observations, which can be confirmed on other insects, is that the oenocytes have become specialized for the production of the lipoproteins of the epicuticle and that when the appropriate time arrives they pass

0.03 mm.

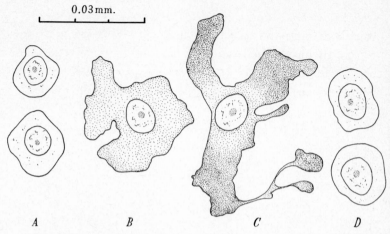

A   B   C   D

Fig. 6. Typical oenocytes below the epidermis in *Rhodnius,* stained with osmic acid and orcein. A, 24 hours after feeding; B, 7 days after feeding; C, 9 days after feeding, just before deposition of the epicuticle; D, 14 days after feeding, just before moulting.

on these materials to the ordinary epidermal cells for secretion on the surface.[93, 95]

We have already mentioned the dermal glands (of which there are, in fact, two distinct kinds in *Rhodnius*). In the most abundant variety the main glandular cell surrounds a vesicle which in the later stages of the moulting process becomes tensely distended with secretion. This is the lipoprotein material which, immediately after moulting, as we have seen, is discharged through the ducts that penetrate the cuticle and spreads out over the surface of the wax and soon hardens to a thin protective covering.[93]

The last components in this system, which we have to mention, are the dermal sense organs that are so characteristic of insects. The hair sensillum is the most familiar type. Like the dermal glands, it also consists of four cells: a trichogen cell which forms the hair; a tormogen cell which surrounds its base and forms the socket; a sense cell which has a distal process running to the base of the hair and a proximal process or axon running to the central nervous system; and, lastly, a neurilemma cell which forms the sheath for the axon (see Fig. 14, p. 36).[101]

These, then, are the chief elements in our drama of growth. The main purpose of this introductory chapter has been to describe their appearance and properties and the parts they play in the actual performance of the functions of "Growth." In the next chapter we shall consider the origin of these component cells and the manner in which they become differentiated one from another.

II · The Capacity for Differentiation

IN the growth of living organisms there are two processes at work: first, the increase in cell number which leads to the progressive enlargement of the body and, second, the differentiation of generalized or embryonic cells to produce all the specialized cell lines which make up the various organs and tissues.

In the development of the embyro the emphasis is largely on differentiation; in postembryonic growth the increase in size is more evident. But the two processes are never wholly separated: so long as growth continues, some degree of differentiation still occurs.

That is very apparent in the epidermis of *Rhodnius*. In the first chapter I sketched in outline the physiological processes which are taking place in the integument of the insect during the moulting cycle, that is, during the period when growth is actually in progress.

For the sake of simplicity I assumed that all the elements which contribute to this process were already present at the outset. But that is not necessarily so: so long as the insect retains the capacity for growth, the epidermis retains a large capacity for differentiation. All the elements that we have described, the oenocytes, the dermal glands, and the dermal sense organs with their sense cells and axons, all these can arise by differentiation from the ordinary epidermal cell. Thus, besides its impressive range of activities in the deposition of the new cuticle, the epidermal cell retains to a substantial degree an embryonic character. That, indeed, is the justification for placing the epidermal cell at the centre of this discussion on growth and form; for this cell is at one and the same time an active agent engaged in the production of form and an embryonic cell with a latent capacity for differentiation. It is a simple model of the embryo.

During the early period of the moulting process, when cell multiplication is taking place, it is possible to observe cell pairs, evidently the daughter cells of a recent cell division, which are a little larger than their neighbours (Fig. 7, A). These pairs of cells enlarge somewhat toward the end of the moulting stage, and they become displaced from the epidermis and join the oenocytes which lie between the epidermal cells and the basement membrane. But they always remain in pairs (Fig. 7, B, C). When the next meal is taken, however, they grow and separate and develop into large oenocytes (Fig. 7, D).[83] Thus a new generation of oenocytes is differentiated from the ordinary epidermal cells during each moulting cycle and joins the existing oenocytes which have survived from the earlier stages and which (like many terminal cell types) seem to be incapable of further multiplication. The factors which regulate this differentiation of new oenocytes from ordinary epidermal cells have not been studied.

A good deal more is known about the differentiation of the sense organs and dermal glands. Each sensory bristle is sur-

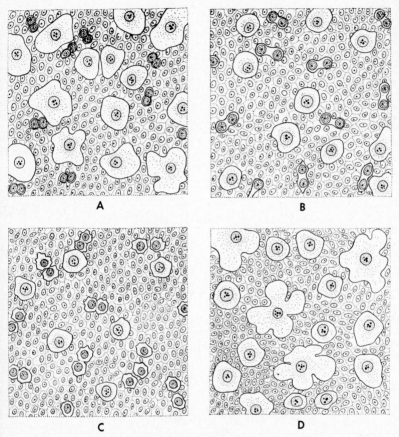

Fig. 7. Stages in the differentiation of oenocytes from the epidermal cells in the 4th-stage larva of *Rhodnius.* A, 10 days after feeding; oenocytes fairly large, new generation of oenocytes in the form of pairs of cells recently differentiated from the epidermis. B, at the time of moulting. C, a week after moulting; previous generation of oenocytes reduced in size, the new generation enlarging but still in pairs. D, 5 days after feeding; old and new generations of oenocytes enlarged and active.

rounded by a smooth "plaque," and beyond this is the ordinary cuticle with its surface thrown into star-shaped folds (Plate II, d). The purpose of that, of course, is to allow for the stretching which follows the ingestion of the enormous meals of blood. Fig. 8, A, shows the general distribution of these organs on the surface of an abdominal segment in a 4th-stage larva. New ones are added at each moult, and it can be seen in

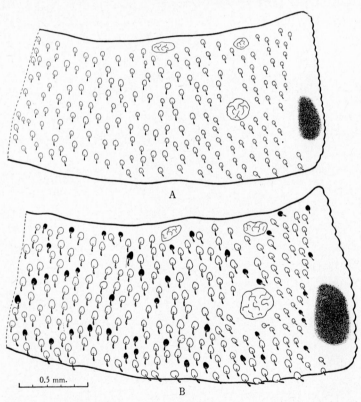

A

0.5 mm.

B

Fig. 8. A, right half of one abdominal tergite in 4th-stage larva of *Rhodnius* showing the sensory hairs and plaques. B, the same after moulting to the 5th stage. The newly developed plaques are shown in black.

Fig. 8, B, that in the 5th stage derived from this particular insect the new plaques, which are shown in black, have appeared at those places where the existing plaques were most widely separated. Two sensory hairs are rarely seen close together; and where there is a wide space devoid of hairs, it will be the site of a new plaque and bristle when the insect moults again.

This suggests that the existing plaques are inhibiting the formation of new plaques in their immediate vicinity, but that when they become separated beyond a certain distance then a new plaque can arise.[88]

It is possible to test this hypothesis experimentally by varying the degree of separation of the plaques.[88] In the newly fed insect the abdomen is tightly distended like a grape; during the next few hours the excess fluid is excreted and the abdomen contracts. If the anus is blocked with paraffin wax immediately after the feed, the distension persists and the plaques are widely separated. The number of new plaques formed can thus be compared in these distended insects, in the normal insects, and in unfed insects with the plaques close together, in which moulting is induced by the introduction of the appropriate hormones. When such an experiment was carried out on a series of 4th-stage larvae, there was no significant difference in the number of new plaques formed in the three groups. The average percentage increase was 26.9 in the insects excreting normally, 26.7 in the insects excessively stretched by blockage of the anus, and 27.4 in the unfed insects.

At first sight these results appear to disprove the influence of mutual separation in determining the appearance of new plaques. But the possibility remains that it is the degree of separation at the preceding moult which is important. This was tested by blocking the anus of the 3rd-instar larvae immediately after feeding, allowing them to moult to the 4th instar, and then feeding them again without occlusion.

When the 3rd-stage larva moults to the 4th stage, there is an average increase of 50.4 per cent in the number of plaques on one segment of the abdomen. Once again there was no difference when the 3rd-stage larva had been stretched by blocking the anus (the average increase was now 46.3 per cent). But there was a striking difference between the two groups at the next moult. In the normal insects there was an average increase of 27.5 per cent when the 4th stage moulted to the 5th stage, whereas in those insects which had been stretched in the 3rd stage there is an increase of 43.8 per cent. Indeed, it was evident on visual inspection that there were more plaques on the group which had been held distended in the 3rd stage.

Similar results can be obtained in a different way. If a heated rod is applied to the cuticle, the cells beneath are killed. The cells around the margin multiply and spread over the wound until a continuous epithelium is restored;[86] and when such an insect moults, it lays down a normal cuticle over the burned area. But this cuticle carries no sensory hairs or plaques. At the next moult, however, new plaques and bristles are formed at more or less regular intervals all over the greater part of this burned area. At the moult after that the regeneration is completed (Fig. 9).[88]

Looking back over these results we may conclude that the closeness of existing plaques or sensilla to one another does control the differentiation of new plaques or sensilla. It appears as though each plaque exerts an inhibitory influence around it and prevents the development of new plaques within a certain radius. It is not, however, the absolute separation of the sensilla that determines the radius over which this influence

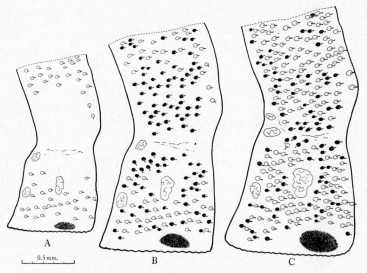

0.5 mm.

A   B   C

Fig. 9. A, left half of third abdominal tergite of 3rd-instar larva of
Rhodnius after a burn in the 2nd instar. B, the same in the 4th instar.
C, the same in the 5th instar. In B and C the newly formed plaques
are shown in black, those appearing at previously existing sites plain.

acts. For the number of new sensilla that appear during moulting is the same whether the insect is unfed and the cuticle not
stretched at all or whether it is stretched to the utmost by
occlusion of the anus after a full meal.

This result suggests that it may be the number of cells
intervening between the sensilla which is important; for in the
early stages of moulting the number is of course the same
whether the insect has been fed or not.

When the stretched insect moults, there is a compensatory
increase in the number of cells in the epidermis, with the result
that when moulting is complete there are the same number of
cells per unit area of cuticle in all the insects; and therefore, in
the insects which had been stretched, the sensilla are separated

by a greater number of cells. For example, in one experiment there was an average of 119 nuclei within the square bounded by four plaques in the normal insect and 148 nuclei in the insect that had been stretched.

If the effective distance between sensilla is to be measured by the number of cells intervening, we should expect to see an increase in the number of new sensilla appearing when these stretched insects moult again. That, as we have found, it what happens.

What is the nature of the inhibitory influence exerted by the sensilla on the surrounding cells? Many kinds of physical and chemical possibilities could be suggested. I personally am attracted by the hypothesis that some chemical constituent in the epidermis is necessary for the differentiation and development of sensilla. The epidermal cells are intimately connected together by filaments which interlace over the surface of the basement membrane, so that there are abundant opportunities for the transmission of materials from cell to cell. According to the hypothesis suggested, as soon as a bristle-forming centre becomes active during moulting, it draws this hypothetical factor from the surrounding cells (Fig. 10). The adjacent cells, drained of this essential element, are therefore incapable of differentiation to form sensilla. Sensillum formation is inhibited. But some cell, sufficiently remote from existing sensilla, becomes active and thus forms a new centre for hair formation which likewise draws the essential element from the zone immediately surrounding it.[88]

This is, of course, merely a working hypothesis, a tool for thought. But in support of it I would point out that all kinds of elements in our society are determined in just this way. A necessary element for the differentiation of a university is a supply of potential students. If these are all drawn off by an

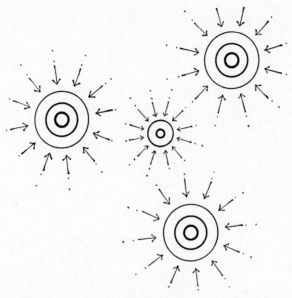

Fig. 10. Diagram to illustrate the hypothesis of the determination of plaques.

existing university, that will inhibit the appearance of another university in the immediate neighborhood. (Of course it is equally possible to suppose that a university gives rise to some product of an offensive nature which inhibits the appearance of another university. It is a matter of personal taste which hypothesis we prefer.)

To return to our sense organs: why are there no new sensilla formed over the healed area at the first moult after a burn? Fig. 11, A, shows the distribution of sensory hairs and plaques in a part of the normal abdomen in *Rhodnius*. The oval bodies are the distended dermal glands. These occur at intervals all over the epidermis, but there is usually a group of four or five clustered round each plaque. Fig. 11, B, shows a correspond-

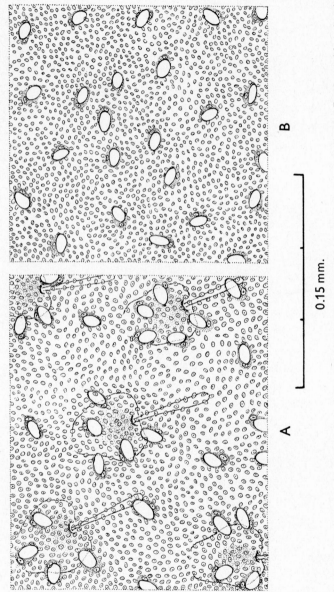

0.15 mm.

Fig. 11. A, epidermis of 4th-stage larva of *Rhodnius* mounted shortly before moulting to the 5th stage, showing the distribution of the plaques and sensory hairs and the distended dermal glands. B, the epidermis of the same insect over an area regenerated after a burn. Dermal glands are present, but no sensory hairs.

ing area on the opposite side of the same insect, where the epidermis had been destroyed by burning. At the first moult after a burn no sensilla and plaques are formed by the newly regenerated epidermis. But, as Fig. 11, B, shows, dermal glands are differentiated within the epidermis, and they are fairly evenly distributed.[101]

As we have seen, the dermal glands are little organs each made up of four cells, just like the sensilla. If dermal glands can be differentiated in the newly formed epidermis why should not sensilla also be differentiated?

I find it tempting to suggest that perhaps the same essential element in the epidermis is needed for the differentiation and development of dermal glands as for sensilla. But perhaps the dermal glands have a lower threshold of response; that is, they require a smaller quantity of this substance. At the first moult after burning there is perhaps sufficient of the hypothetical substance available for the differentiation of dermal glands, but not enough for the differentiation of sensilla. The fact that the dermal glands are less widely spaced than the sensilla could be explained on the basis of this hypothesis.[101]

In short, I am suggesting that an epidermal cell which secures a small amount of the essential factor proceeds to differentiate into a dermal gland, whereas an epidermal cell which secures a large amount can differentiate into a sensillum. This would be an example of a "gradient hypothesis" of the type advocated over many years by C. M. Child.[16] The centre first acquiring the essential factor becomes dominant and produces a gradient in the concentration of this factor in the surrounding zone. It is a necessary part of the gradient hypothesis that quantitative differences of this sort shall result in qualitative differences in the structures produced.

We shall be returning to this point in later chapters, but it may be of interest to indicate here that Locke[42] has recently obtained evidence that there is an anteroposterior gradient of a different kind in each abdominal segment in *Rhodnius,* such that the epidermis at each level unites preferentially with epidermal cells from the same level, which produce a corresponding element in the cuticular pattern.

I would also point out in passing that if this gradient hypothesis for the differentiation of glands and sensilla in the epidermis should prove correct it would provide the basis for a complete theory of differentiation. According to this idea an area in the undifferentiated substrate absorbs and unites with some substance, an "inductor" or "modifier." The cell or plasm thereby becomes determined for some particular type of development (a head, for example), and at the same time, by draining the inductor substance from the surrounding region, it inhibits a similar determination in its vicinity. The zone determined in this way is called a "field." It is immaterial to the argument whether the modified plasma is divided into nucleated cells or whether it forms a nonnucleated continuum.

This process is illustrated in diagrammatic form in Fig. 12. The zone "A" is a "field" determined in this way by the absorption of an inductor. This then proceeds to grow, and within it the same type of change occurs with the uptake of another inductor leading to a new and more specialized "field" of determination "B." And this in turn leads to a new field "C." So the process proceeds, with the uptake by an active centre of the materials necessary for a particular determination and the consequent suppression in the surrounding zones of centres with the same potential activities.

Returning to our *Rhodnius* epidermis, we must now consider what happens to the epidermal cell that has been committed to form either a dermal gland or a sensillum.[101] The first stage

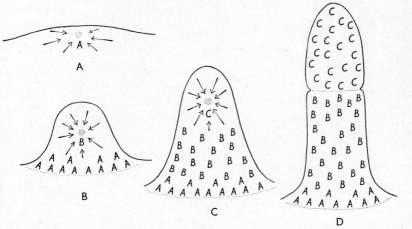

Fig. 12. Stages in the progressive determination of an appendage according to the hypothesis outlined in the text.

at which these organs can be clearly recognized is when they consist of four small cells—presumably the product of two successive divisions in a single epidermal call.

Fig. 13 shows the subsequent stages as these four cells develop into a dermal gland: one nucleus greatly exceeds the others in size and becomes the nucleus of the main gland cell.

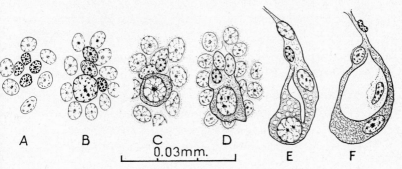

Fig. 13. Stages in the differentiation of a dermal gland in the moulting 4th-stage larva of *Rhodnius.*

[33]

PLATE III

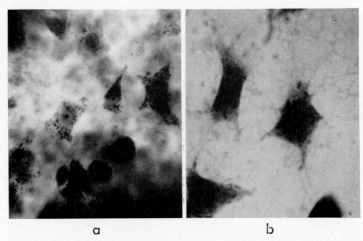

a   b

a, haemocytes with mucopolysaccharide inclusions spread out on the basement membrane. (The epidermal cells are at a lower plane and out of focus.)

b, isolated basement membrane showing haemocytes discharging their contents to add to the substance of the membrane.

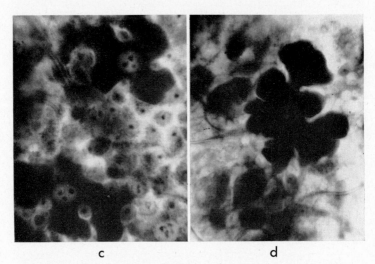

c   d

c, whole mount of epidermis with large lobulated oenocytes.
d, a large oenocyte (epidermis out of focus).

There is one very small nucleus which perhaps forms the sheath of the gland, and two other cells perhaps are concerned in forming the duct.

Fig. 14 shows the corresponding changes in the development of a sensillum. Two cells gradually become very large. One of these is the trichogen cell which sends out a process that develops into the hair; the other is the tormogen cell which forms the socket surrounding the base of the hair and into which the hair is articulated. One cell retains a very small nucleus and becomes the neurilemma cell which provides the sheath for the axon. The fourth cell gives off two processes: one runs to the base of the hair to receive the tactile stimulus when the hair is moved; the other grows inward to the central nervous system and forms the sensory axon.

This axon wanders some little way among the bases of the epidermal cells; but sooner or later it encounters another existing axon or nerve. It immediately allies itself with this and, by following it, finds its way out through the basement membrane into the larger nerves and so eventually into the central nervous system.

It is quite surprising to realize that throughout postembryonic growth in the insect the epidermal cell is still capable of differentiating into nervous tissue which is added to the central nervous system. We are fully justified in claiming that the epidermal cell still retains embryonic powers.

There are several points about this differentiation of sense organs which it is instructive to consider a little more closely. We may consider first the behaviour of the sensory axon. This arises as a filamentous outgrowth from the sense cell. It has no way of knowing where the central nervous system lies. But as soon as it makes contact with another axon or nerve, it becomes associated with it and is thus guided to its destination.

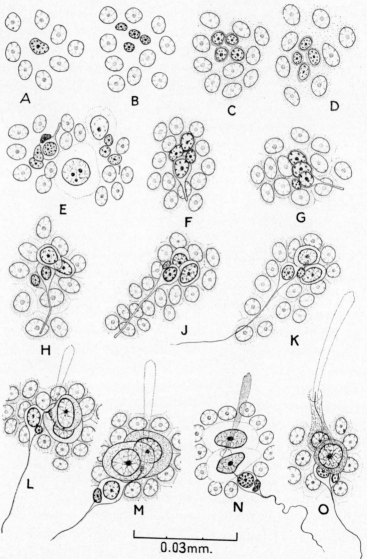

0.03mm.

Fig. 14. Stages in the differentiation of a sensory hair in the 4th-stage larva of *Rhodnius*. (A, B, E, and N stained with Romanes's silver method, the remainder with a modified haematoxylin method.)

That is a general phenomenon in the growth of multicellular animals: each type of cell can recognize its own sort; epithelial cells will associate and join up with epithelial cells, and liver cells with liver cells but not with the cells of other tissues. Indeed, when mixed cells from different species of animals are grown in culture, the mutual affinity of cells from corresponding organs is still evident; thus liver cells of chick and mouse, for example, will aggregate together, but liver cells of the mouse will not associate with lung cells from the same animal.[47]

This class consciousness, this histological clannishness, is one of the guiding principles by which the organization of the body is maintained. But the nature of such mutual affinity is unknown. It may result simply from the physicochemical nature of the cell surfaces, or it may be a more complex interaction, perhaps belonging to the same class as antigen-antibody reactions.

Mutual affinity between cells is well seen during the healing of wounds. If a small incision is made in the integument of *Rhodnius*, the surrounding cells detach themselves from the cuticle and migrate to the margin of the wound. Apparently the injured cells give rise to some substance which "activates" the surrounding cells (just as they become "activated" during the moulting process) and attracts them so that they crowd in upon the wound. But these migrating cells never let go their hold on their neighbours. They may become exceedingly sparse around the wound, but one cell is always connected to another by one or more slender filaments.[86]

If a small square, say 1-2 mm. in width, is excised from the integument, the cells proceed to spread over the wound until they make contact with the epidermal cells advancing inward from the other side, and continuity is restored (Fig. 15). Meanwhile, cell divisions are taking place in the zone where

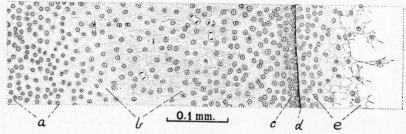

Fig. 15. Epidermis of adult *Rhodnius* 4 days after an excision of the integument about 1 mm. square. *a,* normal unchanged cells; *b,* zone of sparse activated cells, many undergoing division; *c,* zone of congested cells along the margin of the excised area (*d*); *e,* cells spreading over the excised area.

the cells are sparse, and this continues until sufficient new cells have been produced to make good the deficiency.

In this wound-healing process there seem to be two influences at work. Some chemical stimulus from the injured cells activates and attracts the surrounding cells, making them capable of growth and division. And the mutual affinity of the epidermal cells ensures the maintenance of epithelial continuity, leads to the re-establishment of continuity over the wound, and regulates the increase in their numbers so that their proper density is restored.

A curious aberration of this regenerative process is sometimes seen when the axon from a sense cell is cut. The sense cell and its nucleus enlarge as fresh material is passed down the axon; and the axon grows until it meets another axon and by following this reaches the central nervous system again. But sometimes it may fail to make contact with another axon; and eventually it curls round and makes contact with itself. When that happens, it immediately recognizes that this is what it was looking for, and it follows its own tract and grows round and round in circles until a stout circular nerve is developed which never reaches the central nervous system. It forms a kind of neuroma in one plane (Fig. 16).[101]

The normal sensory hairs on the abdomen in *Rhodnius* are regularly oriented in the posterior direction; yet they arise from the differentiation of a single epidermal cell. And when they are regenerated over an extensive burned area, most of the new hairs show the normal orientation. But if a piece of the integument is excised, rotated through 90° or 180° and reim-

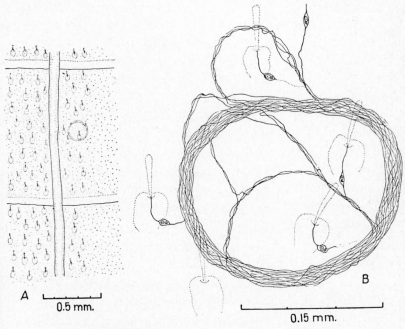

A   0.5 mm.

B   0.15 mm.

Fig. 16. A, low-power view of integument of 4th-stage larva of *Rhodnius* after an extensive burn in the 3rd stage. The burned area lies to the right and is devoid of plaques and hairs. A small "circular nerve" lies just inside the unburned area. B, detail of the "circular nerve," showing the sensory cells from which it is derived.

[39]

planted, the bristles show a corresponding change in orientation at the next moult.[88]

One must therefore conclude that some sort of orientation already exists within the cytoplasm of the undifferentiated epidermal cells, with the result that when they divide to produce the tormogen and trichogen cells these are so placed in respect to one another that the bristles grow out in the predetermined direction.

These observations point to the existence of some kind of "cytoskeleton" within the ordinary epidermal cell, which defines its anteroposterior axis and controls the mutual relations of the daughter cells and in this way the orientation of the resultant structures.

Where the two advancing sheets of epidermal cells come together at the centre of an extensive burn (Fig. 9, C) or at the margin of an implant where the orientation has been reversed, there may be a change in the direction of the sensory hairs. Piepho,[55, 56] who has studied the orientation of scales in displaced implants in Lepidoptera, regards these changes as evidence for some kind of orienting force operating in the general epithelium. I am more inclined to regard them as the result of the rotation or disorientation of epidermal cells in the confused zone where two epidermal sheets are re-establishing continuity. Sometimes, as Locke[42] has recently shown experimentally, disturbances in orientation may be brought about by upsets in the general gradient of the epidermal pattern already mentioned.

Summarizing the arguments presented in this chapter, we may claim to have demonstrated that in addition to the amazing range of physiological activities of which it is capable during the process of moulting and cuticle formation (which were described in Chapter I) the epidermal cell is potentially an embryonic cell, with latent powers of differentiating in several different directions (Fig. 17).

The ordinary epidermal cell may divide to give rise to a pair of oenocytes. It may divide into four and produce a dermal gland cell with the associated cells that form the glandular duct. Or the four daughter cells may differentiate into the bristle-forming and socket-forming cells which give rise to the sensillum and into the sense cell with its neurilemma cell

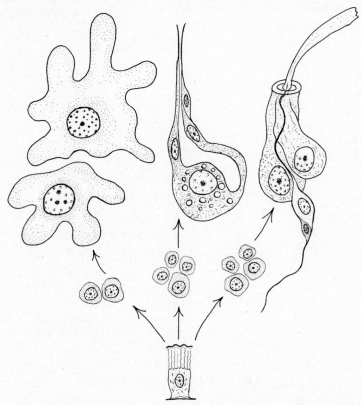

Fig. 17. Diagram summarizing the alternative types of differentiation of the epidermal cell in *Rhodnius*. To the left, differentiation of oenocytes; in the centre, dermal gland; to the right, tactile hair.

both of which grow inwards to become a part of the central nervous system.

Although we have been able to do little more than speculate about the physiological mechanisms which control these processes of differentiation, it is, I hope, evident that we have here a model system which includes in simple outline all the elements that go to compose the differentiated organism. It is a model system on which to study growth. In subsequent chapters we shall see, however, that this brief catalogue by no means exhausts the repertory of this system. The epidermal cell is capable of yet other types of differentiation.

III · Hormones and the
Control of Growth

THUS far our attention has been confined to the growth processes which go forward within the epidermis: the complex sequence of steps that lead up to the formation of a new and larger cuticle at the time of moulting and the processes of differentiation that make possible the appearance of new structures within the epidermis as growth proceeds. We must now consider how these growth changes are initiated and controlled.

In the later years of the last century a number of authors studied the effects of castration and the transplantation of gonads in the insect larva and found that this had no effect on the secondary sexual characters of the adult. These results led to the belief that insects do not secrete hormones. This gratuitous assumption delayed research, and it was not until 1917 that Kopec[40, 41] made the fundamental discovery that pupation in the full-grown caterpillar is brought about by a hormone secreted (as he claimed) by the brain.

That a hormone secreted in the region of the brain induces growth was confirmed in *Rhodnius*: if the *Rhodnius* larva is decapitated within twenty-four hours after feeding it fails to moult, although such headless insects have remained alive for more than a year—much longer, indeed, than if they had been allowed to retain their heads. There is a "critical period" some days after feeding, following which moulting is no longer prevented by decapitation (Fig. 18). The blood now contains the "moulting hormone": if a larva decapitated soon after feeding is joined by means of a capillary tube to a second larva which had been decapitated after the critical period, then the blood of this second larva will cause the first to moult (Plate VI, a).[84, 85]

Similar confirmation was provided by Fraenkel[21] when he showed that the hardening of the larval skin of the blowfly *Calliphora* to form the puparium is due to a hormone produced in or near the anterior ganglionic mass.

At that time (twenty-five years ago) physiologists were reluctant to regard the brain as a secretory organ, and it was at first suggested (without good experimental evidence) that

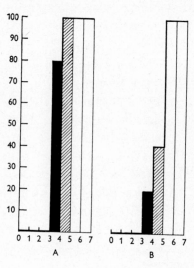

Fig. 18. Histograms to illustrate the "critical period" in the moulting of 4th-stage larvae of *Rhodnius*. Ordinate: percentage of larvae moulting. Abscissa: number of days after feeding, at the time of operation. A, decapitated larvae; B, isolated abdomens.

in *Rhodnius* the corpus allatum, a small endocrine gland which lies immediately behind the brain, might be the source of the moulting hormone.[84]

This idea seemed to gain support from the work of Burtt[11] and Hadorn and Neel[32] who showed that the puparium-forming hormone in the larvae of the flies *Calliphora* and *Drosophila* comes from the ring gland of Weismann, which they regarded as the homologue of the corpus allatum of other insects.

But it was soon found, by Bounhiol[8] in caterpillars and by Pflugfelder[52] in the stick insect *Dixippus*, that moulting would still occur after the corpus allatum had been extirpated. Then Hanström[33] demonstrated the presence of "neurosecretory cells" in the dorsum of the brain in bug *Lygaeus*. I supplied Professor Hanström with *Rhodnius* brains; he confirmed the presence of similar large secretory cells there also; and it was easy to show that the implantation of the region of the brain containing these cells would induce moulting in the decapitated *Rhodnius*, whereas all other regions of the brain were inactive.[89]

Much earlier than this, however, Hachlow[29] had obtained evidence that in Lepidoptera there might be a growth centre of some undetermined nature in the thorax; and in 1940 Fukuda[22] produced conclusive evidence that the immediate source of the moulting hormone in the silkworm is another endocrine gland, the so-called "prothoracic gland" lying in the fat body of the prothorax.

Further study of the ring gland of Weismann in the larva of *Drosophila* and other Diptera showed that this is a composite body (Fig. 19); only the dorsal median part composed of small cells represents the corpus allatum, whereas it is the large lateral cells which are the source of the puparium-

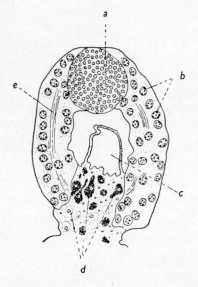

Fig. 19. Section through the ring gland of the young pupa of *Eristalis* (Diptera). (After Cazal, 1948.) *a,* corpus allatum; *b,* large lateral cells ("peritracheal gland"); *c,* aorta; *d,* corpus cardiacum; *e,* nerve to the corpus allatum.

forming hormone,[78] and these cells are now regarded as the homologue of the prothoracic gland.[58, 74]

At this stage, in the early nineteen forties, there appeared to be two equally well-established sources of the "moulting hormone": the neurosecretory cells in the dorsum of the brain and the thoracic glands. These findings were reconciled by Williams[112] in 1947 when he showed that the prothoracic gland in the giant silkworm *Hyalophora cecropia* secretes the growth and moulting hormone only when it is activated by the secretion from the neurosecretory cells of the brain. This two-stage conception of the moulting process is now well established. It has been confirmed in the blowfly *Calliphora,*[58] in *Rhodnius,*[99] in *Sialis,* [60] in *Cephus,* [17] and in other insects.

Fig. 20 shows a typical experiment on *Rhodnius* on the lines first used by Williams in *Hyalophora*. Decapitation at twenty-four hours after feeding prevents moulting. Neurosecretory cells removed from the brain of a moulting larva will cause

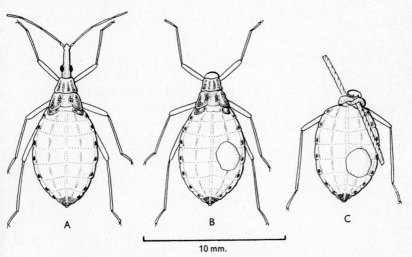

Fig. 20. A, normal 4th-stage larva of *Rhodnius;* B, the same decapitated and with implant in abdomen; C, the same ligatured through metathorax and with implant in the isolated abdomen.

such a decapitated larva to moult, whereas they will not cause moulting in the isolated abdomen. On the other hand, active thoracic glands will induce moulting both in the decapitated larva and in the isolated abdomen.

Under experimental conditions, as we have seen, the neurosecretory cells are active when excised from the brain and implanted elsewhere. But the axons from these cells run to the corpus cardiacum (an organ of nervous origin closely associated with the corpus allatum), and the product of the neurosecretory cells accumulates in the corpus cardiacum and in the dilated endings of these axons (Fig. 21).[34, 52] It is therefore generally assumed that in the normal insect the secretion is liberated from the corpus cardiacum and discharged into the circulating blood.

The stimulus for the liberation of the neurosecretion prob-

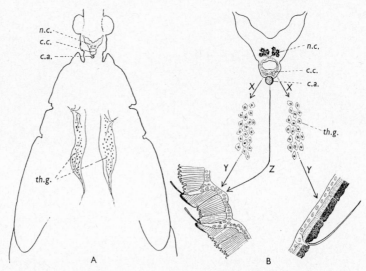

Fig. 21. A, 5th-stage larva of *Rhodnius* showing the location of the chief endocrine organs. B, schema of the endocrine system in *Rhodnius*. *c.a.*, corpus allatum; *c.c.*, corpus cardiacum; *n.c.*, neurosecretory cells; *th.g.*, thoracic gland. *X,* activating hormone from the brain; *Y,* thoracic gland hormone (the moulting hormone "ecdyson"); *Z,* corpus allatum hormone (the juvenile hormone "neotenin"). To the left in B, larval abdominal cuticle is shown; to the right, adult abdominal cuticle.

ably varies in different insects. In *Rhodnius* the stretching of the abdomen by a new meal provides a nervous stimulus to the brain.[84] In the dormant winter pupa of *Hyalophora,* as shown by Van der Kloot,[38] the brain is electrically silent and contains no cholinesterase. When, after prolonged exposure to the winter cold, dormancy comes to an end, electrical activity and cholinesterase reappear; and this is immediately followed by secretory activity in the neurosecretory cells.

Secretion of the brain factor is succeeded by activity in the thoracic glands. Fig. 22, A, shows a part of the thoracic gland

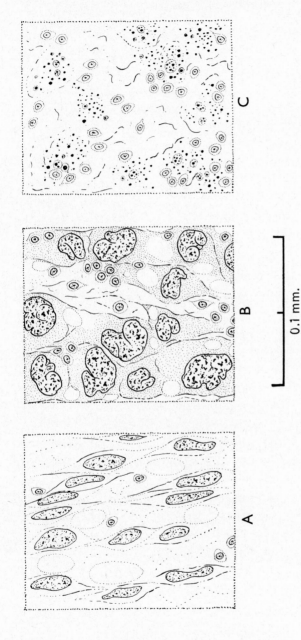

Fig. 22. A, part of thoracic gland in unfed 5th-stage larva of *Rhodnius* showing a few haemocytes; B, the same in 5th-stage larva at 10 days after feeding, show-ing increased numbers of haemocytes; C, the same in adult *Rhodnius* one day after moulting, showing nu-merous haemocytes around the disintegrating nuclei.

0.1 mm.

in the resting larva of *Rhodnius;* the nuclei are small and oval, and there is little visible cytoplasm. Within a few days after feeding, under the action of the brain hormone, the nuclei become greatly enlarged and lobulated and the cytoplasm deeply staining (Fig. 22, B). And then, toward the end of the moulting cycle, these cells revert again to the resting state. They go through these changes during each moult; but after the final moult, when the insect becomes adult, the cells of the thoracic gland break down and disappear so that no further moulting can take place. Fig. 22, C, shows the disintegrating cells in the adult *Rhodnius* twenty-four hours after moulting.[99]

Almost nothing is known yet about the chemical nature of the hormone from the neurosecretory cells. Recently, however, Kobayashi and Kirimura[39] extracted 2 mg. of an oily substance from the brains of 8,500 developing silkworm pupae and found that 0.1 mg. injected into pupae whose development had been arrested by removal of the brain would restore growth and development to the adult moth.

Much more is known about the thoracic gland hormone. The isolation of the active substance which causes hardening in the puparium of the blowfly *Calliphora* was begun in Germany in 1939. Methods for preparing concentrated extracts were gradually worked out by Butenandt and Karlson. Then, a few years ago, these authors found that a substance with the same properties was present in the developing pupa of the commercial silkworm. This made possible a large-scale extraction. Starting with 500 kg. of this material, they were able to isolate in crystalline form some 25 mg. of the active principle, which they term "ecdyson." [13]

This hormone has the empirical formula $C_{18}H_{30}O_4$ and a molecular weight about 300. Ecdyson from the silkworm not only will cause puparium formation in *Calliphora*, but will induce moulting in *Hyalophora* (Williams) and other Lepidoptera and moulting in *Rhodnius*.[105] Since it is effective in the isolated abdomen, it appears to be the active principle of the thoracic gland.

We have now reached a fairly consistent picture of the endocrine organs and hormones regulating growth and moulting in insects. We still need to know far more about the chemistry of these active substances, about the stimuli which regulate their secretion, and about the ways in which they bring about their effects. It is this last topic, the mode of action of the growth hormones in insects, that I propose to consider in this chapter.

The first point to emphasize is that these hormones do not have a sudden or "triggering" effect; they need to act continuously for a considerable period of time. In the resting or dormant insect, in the *Rhodnius* larva, for example, which has completed one moult and awaits another meal to set going a new cycle of growth, the epidermal cells are inactive. The nucleus and nucleolus are small, the cytoplasm attenuated, with little protein or nucleic acid.

Within a few hours after feeding, the epidermal cells are becoming "activated," and by the end of twenty-four hours this change is well advanced; the nuclei, and particularly the nucleoli, are enlarging; the cytoplasm is increasing in amount and becoming rich in protein and nucleic acid. These changes do not occur if the larva is decapitated immediately after feeding: they are not simply the result of nutrition. Indeed, the normal *Rhodnius* larva in the resting phase may have plenty of undigested blood in the stomach.

These results show that the brain factor has been liberated, and the thoracic glands activated, very soon after feeding. But in these same insects (the 4th-stage larvae of *Rhodnius*)

PLATE IV

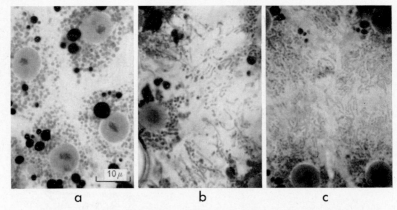

a   b   c

a, fat body cells of *Rhodnius* larva immediately after feeding, showing small nucleoli, fat droplets, and mainly globular mitochondria.

b. fat body cells 24 hours after feeding; nucleoli enlarged; filamentous mitochondria appearing.

c, the same, showing branching filaments among the mitochondria.

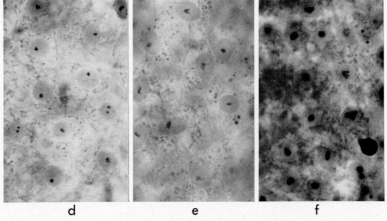

d   e   f

d, epidermal cells of 4th-stage larva in the resting state with small nucleoli and slender mitochondria. (In this and other figures of the epidermis the cuticle lies below the cells and is responsible for the irregular shadows.)

e, the same, 24 hours after injection of ecdyson; nucleoli enlarged and mitochondria swollen.

f, the same, at 2 days after feeding. Mitochondria greatly swollen; further enlargement of nucleoli.

PLATE IV—*Continued*

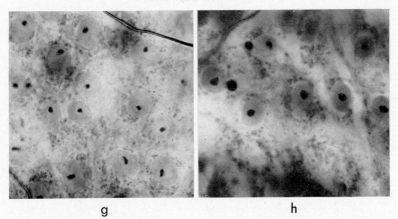

g   h

g, epidermal cells in adult *Rhodnius,* normal resting state. Nucleoli and mitochondria relatively small.

h, the same, in the vicinity of a minute incision. Nucleoli much enlarged; mitochondria swollen and many of them oriented in the direction of the wound below and to the right.

decapitation will prevent moulting even when carried out as late as two and a half to three days after feeding (Fig. 18). What the brain factor is doing during this period is not known. Perhaps it is contributing some component that is essential for the formation of ecdyson by the thoracic gland.

More is known about the action of the thoracic gland hormone. It appears to act directly on the cells that are to be caused to grow; or, at least, no intermediate steps have yet been discovered. The *Rhodnius* larva may be well nourished, with blood in process of digestion in the stomach, and yet it fails to grow until the neurosecretory cells are stimulated to discharge their hormone by the insect's taking a large meal of blood. This phenomenon, of an organism that is living and yet fails to grow, is common enough in animals and plants. It is seen in dormant seeds, in unfertilized eggs, in insects during hibernation or diapause. In fact, it was pointed out many years ago[84] that the *Rhodnius* larva which was well nourished, but whose endocrine system was inactive, so that no moulting hormone was present in the blood, was in a state of diapause. This interpretation suggested that the immediate cause of diapause in other insects was probably a temporary absence of growth hormones.

But that does not tell us what the hormones are doing, or what is the nature of the deficiency in these insects when the hormones are absent. It was suggested at one time by Runnström[62] that the deficiency in the unfertilized egg was a lack of cytochrome. Bodine and his school took up this idea in studying diapause in the egg of the grasshopper *Melanoplus*. But they failed to find any clear correlation between the intensity of respiration and the amount of cytochrome oxidase;[7,2] it appeared that some other component of the cytochrome system was the variable factor.

It has long been known that during the pupal stage of insects the consumption of oxygen is at first high; it then falls to a low level, which is maintained during diapause, and finally rises steeply as development proceeds before emergence. It was shown by Wolsky[118] and others that the course of this curve was correlated with the amount or the activity of the Warburg-Keilin system of respiratory enzymes and with the amount of the various substrate-dehydrogenase systems.

Williams and his colleagues have gone much further along these lines.[113, 114] They showed that during diapause the pupa of the giant silk moth *Hyalophora* is almost completely insensitive to cyanide and other poisons acting on the cytochrome system, whereas the growing larva and the actively developing pupa are highly sensitive. During diapause, cytochrome oxidase is present in some quantity, but cytochrome C appears to be virtually absent from most of the tissues; it reappears in notable amounts very rapidly when growth is renewed.

From these observations, which have been worked out in great detail, Williams draws the conclusion that the essential metabolic deficiency in the diapausing pupa is a lack of cytochrome C and that the action of the hormone of the thoracic gland is to "preside over the synthesis of cytochrome C."

The study of this question in *Rhodnius* has led to a somewhat different way of looking at the problem. During the resting stage between moults, the larva of *Rhodnius*, unlike the pupa of *Hyalophora*, is actively motile. It has a large amount of muscle in the legs and thorax which contains a great quantity of active cytochrome. And yet, in the absence of the moulting hormone, these insects do not grow.

If *Rhodnius* larvae are placed individually in a respirometer, it is possible to follow the course of oxygen uptake during the moulting cycle (Fig. 23). This is low in the unfed insect. After feeding, it rises steadily for about five days and then remains

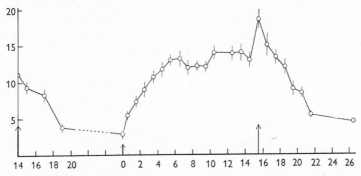

Fig. 23. Oxygen uptake during the moulting cycle in the 4th-stage larva of *Rhodnius*. Ordinate: oxygen consumption as mm.^{3} per insect per hour. Abscissa: days after feeding. The short arrow marks the time of feeding, the long arrows the times of moulting.

more or less constant until it commonly rises to a peak at the time of moulting. During the next five or six days respiration falls gradually to a new low level.

Abundant cytocrome is present in the muscles of the resting insect; yet the rate of respiration is very low. That, of course, is because the insect rests practically motionless in the respirometer. Only for that reason is it possible to observe the effects of growth and moulting upon the course of oxygen uptake.

This is a point of some importance, obvious though it is. The oxygen consumption of an animal is determined not by the amount of oxidizing enzymes present, but by the functional activity of the body. On the other hand, if the demand of the body for oxygen increases, we may expect the amount of oxidizing enzymes likewise to increase in order to meet the need. To attribute increased respiration to an increased supply of enzymes, as is sometimes done,[1] is to underestimate the capacity of the organism to regulate its own metabolism. During the early stages of embryonic development in *Tubifex,* for example, the rate of oxygen consumption increases twentyfold, whereas the activity of cytochrome oxidase shows no definite change. Clearly, at the outset of development only a small fraction of the capacity of the system is employed.[79]

We must now determine what are the visible effects taking place in the cells under the action of the moulting hormone. Either we can observe these changes as they occur normally in *Rhodnius* larvae after feeding or, in order to separate the effects of nutrition alone, we can decapitate the larvae soon after feeding and then inject half of them with ecdyson in Ringer's solution and the other half with Ringer's solution alone.

Three tissues have been selected for study: the fat body, the ventral abdominal muscles, and the epidermis of the abdomen.[109] The fat body is actively engaged in all kinds of syntheses throughout the moulting cycle. In the later stages particularly, it accumulates large amounts of fat, glycogen, and protein for rapid transfer to the growing tissues.

Plate IV, *a*, shows the fat body in the resting or newly fed insect: the nuclei have relatively small nucleoli, and the mitochondria are mostly coccoid or oval in form with a few short rods. Within six hours after feeding, or injection of ecdyson, there is a detectable increase in ribonucleic acid around the nuclei of these cells. Within twenty-four hours after feeding, the nucleoli are greatly enlarged and lobulated (Plate IV, *b*, *c*); much nucleic acid is accumulating; the mitochondria appear to be increasing in number; there are many filamentous forms which seem to be radiating from the nucleus and many of them are branching.

The second tissue is the ventral abdominal group of muscles which in *Rhodnius* undergo a remarkable cycle during each moulting stage.[107] They are fully formed only at the time of moulting, when they are needed to furnish the hydraulic pressure in the blood that is used to split the old cuticle and to expand the appendages (p. 12). They show up brilliantly when the sternites of the newly moulted larva are examined in polarized light. By three days after moulting they can be seen only as "ghosts" running across the segments. By five days the birefringent fibrils have disappeared completely; nothing remains but the muscle sheath, containing the nuclei and a very little cytoplasm. The insect has now loosened its belt, and the abdomen is ready to receive the next enormous meal of blood.

The same thing happens at the time of hatching from the egg. Plate V, *a*, shows the ventral muscles immediately after hatching; three days later they have disappeared (Plate V, *b*). They are re-formed after feeding (Plate V, *c-e*): by four days

PLATE V

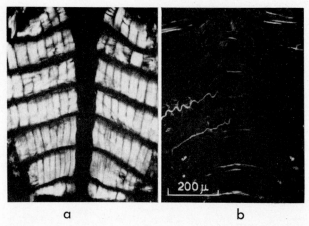

a   b

a, sternites of abdomen of newly hatched larva of *Rhodnius*, seen in polarized light to show the ventral muscles.

b, the same, 3 days after hatching; the muscles have disappeared.

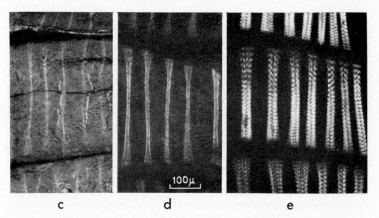

c   d   e

c, sternal muscles in 1st-stage larva 4 days after feeding. (Polarized light.)

d, the same at 5 days after feeding; striation appearing.

e, the same at 10 days after feeding; muscles fully formed.

[58]

PLATE V—*Continued*

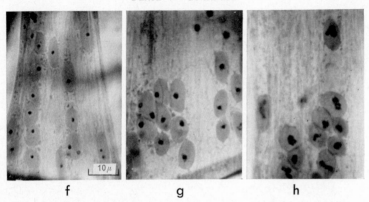

f   g   h

f. ventral abdominal muscle of 4th-stage larva in resting state show-ing small nuclei and nucleoli and mitochondria. (Whole mount stained with osmium-ethyl gallate.)

g, the same at one day after feeding; nuclei, nucleoli, and mito-chondria enlarging.

h, the same at 3 days after feeding; further enlargement of nuclei and nucleoli; abundant mitochondria.

after feeding birefringent fibrils have reappeared; by five days striation is beginning to appear; by the time of the next moult the muscles are fully formed again.

Fig. 24 shows the same cycle of changes in the 1st- and 2nd-stage larvae as seen in stained preparations, and Plate V, *f-h,* shows the changes in the nuclei and mitochondria during the first three days after feeding in the 4th-stage larva. In the resting state or in the newly fed insect (Plate V, *f*) the nuclei and nucleoli are small and the mitochondria small and few in number. By one day after feeding (Plate V, *g*) nuclei and nucleoli are enlarging, the mitochondria are swollen and in-creasing in number, and ribonucleic acid in the cytoplasm is increasing. By three days after feeding (Plate V, *h*) the nu-cleoli are enormously enlarged; mitochondria are now very

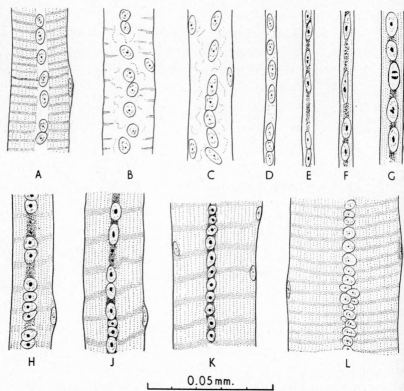

Fig. 24. Changes in the abdominal muscles of the 1st-stage larva after hatching and after feeding. A, immediately after hatching (cf. Plate V,a). B, 2 days after hatching. C, 4 days after hatching (cf. Plate V,b). D, 14 days after hatching, immediately after feeding. E, 2 days after feeding. F, 4 days after feeding (cf. Plate V,c). G, 5 days after feeding (cf. Plate V,d). H, 6 days after feeding. J, 7 days after feeding. K, 9 days after feeding (cf. Plate V,e). L, 11 days after feeding (newly moulted 2nd-stage larva).

numerous, and many of them are elongated longitudinally. The muscle fibrils, not visible in the photograph, are now beginning to separate out between these rows of mitochondria.

The epidermis shows comparable changes[109]. Plate IV, d,

shows the epidermis of an insect decapitated immediately after feeding, injected with Ringer's solution, and mounted twenty-four hours later. The nucleoli are small, the mitochondria mostly in the form of minute granules or slender filaments. That represents the resting state. Plate IV, *e*, shows epidermal cells in a similar insect twenty-four hours after the injection of ecdyson. The nucleoli are enlarging, and the mitochondria are for the most part contracted and swollen to form rounded or oval bodies. Ribonucleic acid (not visible in these preparations) is increasing markedly in the cytoplasm. These changes are already becoming evident within six hours after the injection of ecdyson.

Plate IV, *f*, shows the epidermal cells two days after feeding or ecdyson injection. The nucleoli are still further enlarged, the mitochondria are increasing in number, and the cells are thickening so that in these whole mounts the mitochondria now form a rather confused mass. By four days the cells form a cubical epithelium; they are loaded with protein and nucleic acid, the nucleoli are lobulated and branched, and mitosis is beginning.

Preliminary study with the electron microscope showed that in the resting epidermal cell the mitochondria have an average diameter of 0.15 μ. Within six hours after the injection of ecdyson the globular mitochondria have an average thickness of 0.28 μ. At nine days after feeding, at the height of cuticle formation, the cells are filled with a dense ergastoplasm or laminated endoplasmic reticulum rich in ribonucleic acid, which largely obscures the abundant mitochondria.

In each of these tissues, fat body, muscles, and epidermis, the essential changes are the same. There is a great enlargement of the nucleolus and an increase in the ribonucleoprotein in the cytoplasm. These changes begin within an hour or two after feeding. They are followed, at a comparatively late stage (four or five days after feeding), by mitosis and the deposition of the specific products of the cells (muscle fibrils, cuticle, and so on).

The difference between the resting cell and the cell activated by the moulting hormone seems to lie in the restoration of the capacity for protein synthesis in the activated cells. Protein synthesis is not a simple reversal of peptide hydrolysis; it is an endothermic process which requires large amounts of energy. There are, of course, many other synthetic processes going on when growth begins, notably, the oxidative deamination of amino acids, with the deposition of reserves of fat and glycogen; but the most important from a quantitative point of view is the synthesis of nucleic acids and protein.

I would suggest that the characteristic defect in the resting or dormant insect, where no moulting hormone is being secreted, is a failure of protein synthesis and that the curve of respiration during moulting (Fig. 23) is very largely a measure of the activity of protein synthesis. There are the rapid rise as the nucleic acid and protein in the cytoplasm are increased during the first few days, the sustained high level as new cells, muscle fibrils, and cuticle are formed, the continuing high level after moulting as more protein and chitin are added to the cuticle, and the gradual fall to the resting level as this process comes to an end about six or seven days after moulting.

Among the most important types of protein that are synthesized when growth begins will be enzymes. These will catalyze further growth, so that in this sense growth is an autocatalytic process. It had often been noted in *Rhodnius* that in the decapitated insect digestion of the blood meal is markedly delayed. Whether the more active digestion in the normal insect was a direct effect of the growth and moulting hormone or whether it was a secondary consequence of the increasing demands of the growing tissues was not apparent. Recently, however, it has been shown experimentally by Ellen Thomsen and Ib Möller[75] that in the adult blowfly *Calliphora* the secretion of the neurosecretory cells causes an increase in the production of proteolytic enzymes by the gut. It is likely that the growth and moulting hormone has the same effect and that this particular form of protein synthesis will have far-reaching "catalytic" effects on nutrition and growth throughout the body.

We can only speculate as to how the moulting hormone restores the capacity for protein synthesis[109]. According to current conceptions the energy necessary for the process is provided in the form of adenosine triphosphate (ATP) produced by cycles of oxidative phosphorylation in the mitochondria and fed into the enzyme system which links the amino acids together.

It is possible to imagine many points at which the chain of reactions leading to protein synthesis might be interrupted in the absence of the growth and moulting hormone. Williams[113] had suggested that the key point is the lack of cytochrome C in the energy-producing cycle of the mitochondria. I personally favour the hypothesis that the complete enzyme system may often be present in the cells even in the resting state, but that the protein-synthesizing enzymes are segregated from their substrates.*

Since we are almost completely ignorant of how chemical processes in living cells are controlled and directed, it is impossible to express a hypothesis of this kind in any but the

* Shappirio and Williams[73] have found that even in the Cecropia silkworm cytochrome C is present, albeit in small amounts only, during diapause. They are now inclined to regard the "synthesis of cytochromes b and C as reactions which intervene between the primary action of the hormone and the insect's developmental response."

vaguest of terms. But it is quite evident that the enzymes in the cell must normally be largely insulated from their substrates. That is one of the conditions of life. Were that not so, the body would autolyze and die within a few moments. We may picture the "growth and moulting hormone" as being concerned in regulating the transport of materials within the cell; that is, it may control the activity of the synthetic system of the cell by regulating permeability relations or transport mechanisms.

This conception is an old one in biology. It was suggested many years ago by Loeb[43] that artificial parthenogenesis in the egg of echinoderms or amphibia results from a partial cytolysis within the cell. Holtfreter[36] has put forward the hypothesis that the activation of the blastoderm which precedes neural plate formation in vertebrates is likewise a consequence of a "sublethal cytolysis." And Runnström[63] suggests that the initiation of development in the egg may be due to the activation of various enzymes.

In the adult *Rhodnius,* in the absence of the moulting hormone, the epidermal cells are permanently in the resting state, with small nucleoli and relatively small and slender mitochondria (Plate IV, *g*). But if the epidermis is cut with a knife, the injured cells undergo autolysis, and they give rise to products which diffuse into the surrounding zone and activate the surrounding cells (p. 38).[86]

Plate IV, *h,* shows the epidermal cells in the neighborhood of an incision, twenty-four hours after the injury. The cut itself in this experiment was very superficial, not even passing through the basement membrane. It lies about 180 μ, about fifteen cell widths, below and to the right of the cells illustrated. Within twenty-four hours the cells around the wound, up to a distance of 240 μ, showed great enlargement of the nucleoli, the mitochondria were swollen and globular or elongated and oriented toward the wound, and the cytoplasm was filled with ribonucleoprotein.[109]

These changes in the epidermal cells are indistinguishable from those which are seen in the early stages of normal moulting. Whether there is any relation between the products of autolysis in the injured cells which cause this wound reaction and the moulting hormone which causes the very similar general reaction throughout the body remains to be seen.

IV ✦ Hormones and the Control of Form

THE physiological activities of the epidermal cell during the course of growth and differentiation and cuticle formation have now been considered, as well as the stimulation of these activities by the thoracic gland hormone or in response to local injury. But one of the most striking characteristics of the epidermal cell of the insect is its capacity for laying down cuticle of exceedingly diverse types at successive stages in its life cycle. It is this capacity which forms the basis of the metamorphosis from larva to pupa and imago that is so conspicuous in the holometabolous insects.

In a hemimetabolous insect such as *Rhodnius,* where the mode of life is the same at all stages of the life cycle, the general build of the animal remains unchanged from larva to adult. But that does not alter the fact that in *Rhodnius,* also, there is a clear-cut "metamorphosis" (Plate I). Throughout the first five moulting stages the wing lobes and the developing genitalia are inconspicuous. At the final moult large membranous wings are formed, the whole structure of the thorax is correspondingly altered, elaborate external genitalia are differentiated, ocelli appear for the first time, and complicated adhesive or climbing organs are developed on the first two pairs of legs.

For our present purpose it will be convenient to concentrate mainly upon the changes that occur at metamorphosis in the general structure of the abdomen (Fig. 25). During the larval stages the cuticle is relatively thick; it is highly extensible, for the epicuticle is thrown into deep stellate folds and has no thick sclerotized exocuticle save at the smooth rounded plaques,

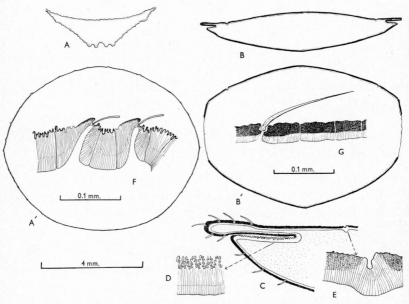

Fig. 25. A, transverse section of abdomen of unfed 5th-stage larva of *Rhodnius.* A', the same immediately after feeding. B, transverse section of abdomen of unfed adult. B', the same immediately after feeding. C, detail of lateral pleat in abdomen of unfed adult. D, detail of extensible lower wall of this pleat. E, detail of "hinge line" in tergites. F, longitudinal section of abdominal tergite of 5th-stage larva. G, longitudinal section of abdominal tergite of adult.

each bearing a bristle, which are scattered regularly over the surface.

In the adult, the surface of the cuticle is thrown mainly into transverse folds; it is much thinner than in the larval stages, but the outer half is sclerotized to form a hard exocuticle so that it is inextensible. There are few bristles (except at the sides of the abdomen) and no plaques. The distension of the abdomen is provided for, not by a general stretching of the cuticle, but by the unfolding of a lateral pleat and the elasticity of a lateral strip of soft cuticle.[83]

Fig. 26 shows for comparison a view of the upper surface

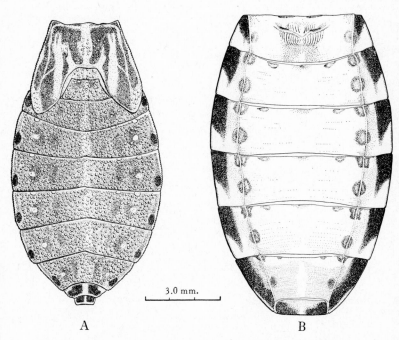

3.0 mm.

A   B

Fig. 26. A, dorsal view of meso- and metathorax and abdomen of 5th-stage larva of *Rhodnius;* B, dorsal view of abdomen of adult female.

of the abdomen in the 5th-stage larva and the adult. Apart from the differences just noted, attention may be directed to the small rounded pigment spots in the larva, which lie at the posterior angle of each segment; in the adult there is a large trapezoidal spot at the anterior angle of each segment. One should note also the parallel ridges in the central region of the fused first and second segments of the adult. In addition, the adult shows a line of soft cuticle passing through the muscle insertions some distance from the lateral margin. This is the so-called "hinge line" along which the dorsal cuticle bends when the abdomen is distended by a meal (Fig. 25 C, E).

All these changes, taken together, are actually more extensive than those which occur in the abdomen of many holometabolous insects, such as Coleoptera or Lepidoptera, at the time of metamorphosis to the pupa.

In holometabolous or "endopterygote" insects, those groups of epidermal cells which are destined to form certain of the imaginal structures, such as wings, take no part in the deposition of cuticle during the larval stages. These cells are invaginated to form small pockets and are then evaginated within these pockets without appearing externally (Fig. 27). It is not until the pupal moult that these lobes become everted and visible and take part in the formation of the cuticle. By means of this arrangement some of the more elaborate adult structures, such as the wings, can make a considerable amount of growth without having to take part in the ordinary business of cuticle formation during each larval moult.

But even in Lepidoptera and Coleoptera this segregation of imaginal cells in the form of the so-called "imaginal discs" affects only certain parts of the body. Throughout the greater part of the body, in the abdomen, for example, the epidermal cells that have been depositing the larval cuticle now change

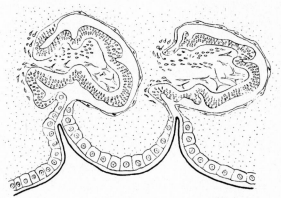

Fig. 27. Longitudinal section through the imaginal discs of the wings in full-grown larvae of an ant (after Pérez).

their activities and proceed to lay down pupal and adult cuticle. In other words, the characteristic of metamorphosis in insects is not the activation of the dormant imaginal discs, but the changed functions of the ordinary epidermal cells.

Since the epidermal cells which secrete the adult cuticle are the same cells as have previously laid down the larval cuticle or are the direct descendants of these cells, it is obvious that the capacity to lay down either larval or adult cuticle is latent within the selfsame cell.

This is strikingly illustrated during the repair of injuries. The pattern of the body surface results from the fact that the underlying epidermal cells have become determined to lay down cuticle of some characteristic type: some to form black pigmented cuticle, others brown sclerotized cuticle, and yet others soft and colourless cuticle.

During the repair of a burn, when the cells at the margin of the injury divide and migrate inward until continuity is restored, they carry with them their special characteristics. Thus,

[71]

if the burn has passed through a couple of black pigment spots, when the insect lays down a new cuticle and moults, the regenerated zone will show two black sectors continuous with these spots (Fig. 28). Other elements in the pattern show the same centripetal displacement.[89]

Similarly, if a small burn is inflicted between two lateral pigment spots in the 3rd-instar larva, these will be found united to form a continuous spot in the 4th and 5th stages. Or if one pigment spot is burned out, its place will be taken by unpigmented cuticle at the next instar (Fig. 29, B).

Now it so happens that in the *Rhodnius* adult (Fig. 26) the black pigment spots at the margin of the tergites occupy the

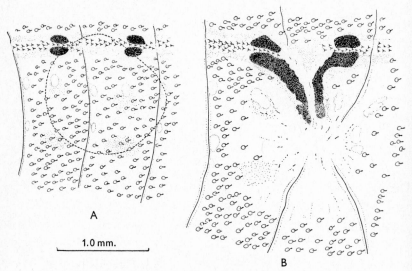

A

1.0 mm.

B

Fig. 28. A, lateral region of the dorsal surface of two segments in a 3rd-stage larva of *Rhodnius* showing the double row of marginal plaques above, and beyond this a small piece of the ventral surface. The broken line shows the extent of the epidermis killed by burning. B, the corresponding region in the 4th-stage larva after healing and moulting.

[72]

anterior angle of each segment which was unpigmented in the larva, whereas the oval area at the posterior angle which was pigmented in the larva is now colourless. Consequently, when the insects described in the last experiment undergo metamorphosis to the adult, the effects on the pigment pattern are reversed: where two black pigment spots had united in the larva, there is an almost unpigmented zone in the adult; and where a pigment spot had been eliminated in the larva, two adjacent pigment spots of the adult have become fused (Fig. 29, C).[89]

Likewise, at the anterior end of the abdomen in the adult, that is, on the first and second tergites, there is the characteristic pattern of ridged brown cuticle. There is no sign of this structure in the larva; and after an extensive burn in this

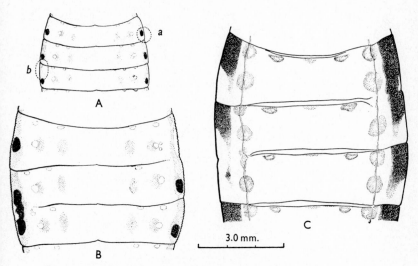

Fig. 29. A, third, fourth and fifth tergites of a normal 3rd-stage larva of *Rhodnius*. The broken lines at *a* and *b* show the regions burned. B, corresponding segments in the 5th-stage larva resulting. C, corresponding segments in the adult resulting.

[73]

region the cuticle pattern shows no very obvious distortion. But when such an insect undergoes metamorphosis to the adult, this ridged cuticle shows a striking displacement (Fig. 30).

These results serve to emphasize that the adult pattern is already latent within the larval cells and that, when these cells divide, the capacity to form particular elements in this pattern is transmitted to the daughter cells. They carry their properties with them through their divisions and wanderings, but these properties remain latent until metamorphosis occurs. One gets the impression that the organism is made up of competing communities of cells, the normal body pattern being maintained by the population pressure of these jostling communities.

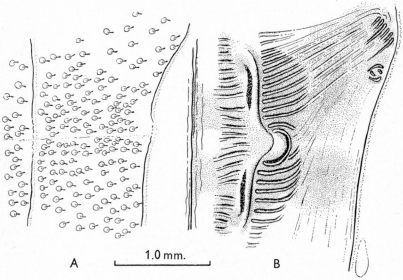

1.0 mm.

A   B

Fig. 30. A, part of the mid-dorsal region of the first and second segments in a 5th-stage larva of *Rhodnius* which had been burned on the right side in the 3rd stage. B, corresponding segments in the adult resulting.

[74]

From these observations one could infer that, if the appropriate conditions were provided, the cells could realize their latent imaginal characters, and metamorphosis could take place at any period in larval growth. With certain limitations that has proved to be the case.

The first indication of this was given when larvae of *Rhodnius* were decapitated at different times after feeding. If the head was removed before the "critical period" (see p. 44), moulting failed to occur at all; and if decapitation was in the late stages, a normal larval cuticle was laid down. But there is a time, just shortly after the critical period, when decapitation is followed by moulting, but the new cuticle, instead of being of larval type, shows adult characters (Fig. 31). Decapitation has resulted in precocious metamorphosis.[84]

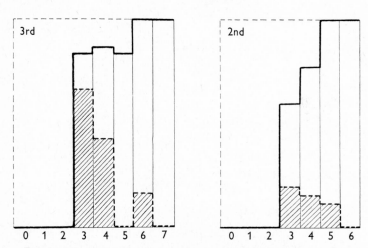

Fig. 31. Chart showing the proportion of *Rhodnius* larvae in the 3rd and 2nd stage which moulted, out of batches decapitated at different times after feeding. Figures on the base line represent days after feeding. The uppermost level represents 100 per cent moulting. The broken line (above shaded area) shows the proportion of insects developing adult characters.

Clearly, the head is preventing the occurrence of metamorphosis. The action was evidently hormonal in nature, for if a 4th-stage larva with the head intact (except for removal of its extreme tip) was joined to a decapitated 5th-stage larva, this did not undergo metamorphosis, but developed larval characters again when it moulted (Fig. 32).

The source of this hormone was soon traced to the corpus allatum, a small gland of internal secretion lying immediately behind the brain in close relation with the corpus cardiacum (Fig. 21). If a 4th-stage larva with the brain removed but the corpus allatum intact was joined shortly after the "critical period" to a 4th-stage larva decapitated at one day after feeding, the latter was caused to moult once more into a larva; whereas if the corpus allatum was absent from the first insect, the second underwent metamorphosis. It is of interest to note in passing that when these insects are joined together the epidermis unites so that it is impossible to say where one individual ends and the other begins. That is equally true when two species are concerned, such as *Rhodnius* and *Triatoma* or *Rhodnius* and *Cimex*.

If the corpus allatum is transplanted from a 4th-stage larva

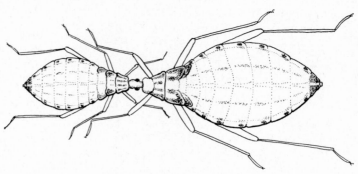

Fig. 32. Larva at earlier stage, with the tip of the head removed (to the left), joined to a decapitated larva at later stage (to the right).

into the abdomen of a 5th-stage larva, the latter fails to undergo metamorphosis when it moults, but again develops larval characters: it becomes a giant or 6th-stage larva, (Plate VI, *b*). Sometimes the results are less complete than that, and forms with larval abdomens but intermediate wings are produced. Or they might develop into normal adults with a diffuse area of larval cuticle on the abdomen; and sometimes there is nothing to see but a tiny patch of larval cuticle immediately overlying the implanted corpus allatum, proving that the hormone exerts its action directly upon the epidermal cells (Plate VIII, *b*).[85]

In the 5th-stage larva the situation is changed. The corpus allatum appears completely normal, but it will no longer prevent metamorphosis when transplanted into another 5th-stage larva. And if a 1st-stage larva recently hatched from the egg is decapitated with removal of the corpus allatum and is then joined to the tip of the head of a moulting 5th-stage larva (Plate VI, *c*), it is caused to moult but it develops adult characters: the adult pattern, rudimentary genitalia, and the rudiments of wings (see Fig. 38, p. 93).

On the other hand, soon after the insect has become adult, the corpus allatum again becomes active, and the gland removed from a mature adult and implanted into a 5th-stage larva will once more lead to the arrest of metamorphosis and the production of a 6th-stage larva. Even a 7th-stage larva has been produced by further implantations into a 6th stage. In the adult insect the normal function of the corpus allatum secretion is different: it is necessary in the female for the full development of the eggs, with the deposition of yolk; and it has some small effects on the accessory glands of the male.[85]

A similar action of the corpus allatum in delaying the occurrence of metamorphosis has been confirmed in most groups of

PLATE VI

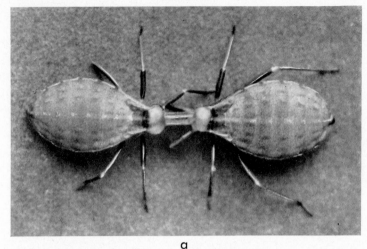

a

a, 4th-stage larva decapitated after the critical period and joined by means of a capillary tube to a 4th-stage larva decapitated at one day after moulting.

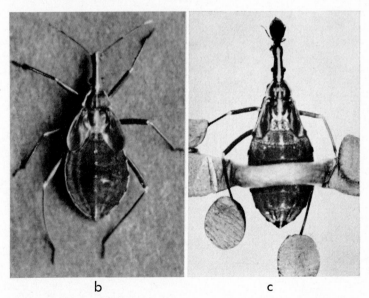

b   c

b, giant or 6th-stage larva of *Rhodnius* produced by implanting the corpus allatum of a 4th-stage larva into the abdomen of the 5th stage.

c, moulting 5th-stage larva with a decapitated 1st-stage larva joined to the tip of the head.

insects, and the active principle is either identical in all or at least sufficiently similar for the corpus allatum to be effective after transfer from one order to another. Sixth-stage larvae of *Rhodnius,* for example, can be produced by implantation of corpora allata from the adult cockroach (*Periplaneta*) into 5th-stage larvae.[49, 100] And implantation of the corpus allatum from the larva of the blowfly *Calliphora,* although it has not produced this general effect, has led to the appearance of a local patch of unmistakable larval cuticle over the implanted gland.[102]

Attempts to extract the corpus allatum hormone were for long unsuccessful. It appears from recent experiments that only minute traces are present in the blood and tissues at any moment.[111] But the corpus allatum, as already brought out, regains its activity in the adult of both sexes. That is so also in the giant silk moth *Hyalophora cecropia.* In the female Cecropia moth there do not seem to be excessive quantities of the hormone in the tissues, but it has been shown by C. M. Williams that in the abdomen of the male large amounts of the hormone do accumulate, apparently stored in the tissue fats. These fats can be extracted with ether to give an active hormone preparation, and this will bring about the same retention of larval characters in all the insects tested—in *Hyalophora* and *Pieris* (Lepidoptera), in *Tenebrio* (Coleoptera), in *Rhodnius* (Hemiptera)—as does the implantation of a living corpus allatum.[115]

We saw that this hormone acts directly upon the epidermal cells. The active extract can be applied to them from outside. It does not readily pass through the uninjured cuticle; but if the impermeable layer of cement and wax is removed by abrasion (for example, by allowing a suspension of crystalline alumina to dry on the surface[110]), it is possible to make local applications to sharply defined areas and thus to produce localized patches of larval cuticle in an otherwise adult insect. Plate VII, *b,* shows a single larval segment interposed in the abdomen of an adult *Rhodnius;* in Plate VII, *c,* a part of the abdomen of an adult *Rhodnius* has been engraved with larval cuticle; Plate VII, *a,* shows a *Rhodnius* adult with a larval wing lobe following the local application of the extract.[111]

It was shown some years ago[89] that the different elements in the cuticle pattern remain susceptible to the hormone for different periods, and this can be readily confirmed by means of local applications of the active extract. For example, if the 5th-stage larva of *Rhodnius* is allowed to develop toward the adult for nine days after feeding and then the hormone is applied to the epidermal cells, the resulting cuticle shows the normal star-shaped folding of the surface that is characteristic of the larva. The bristles and plaques have disappeared (the hormone has been applied too late to save them), but the sites previously occupied by plaques can be recognized because the cuticle in these regions lacks the usual dark grey pigment. This experiment is of some interest since it shows that the different capacities of a given cell, which contribute to the general pattern, can be determined to some extent independently of one another.

We must now consider the mode of action of the corpus allatum hormone upon the epidermal cell. When its effects were first discovered, it was described as preventing the realization of adult characters and thus inhibiting metamorphosis. It was therefore called the "inhibitory hormone"; and in the second paper devoted to the control of metamorphosis in *Rhodnius*[85] an attempt was made to describe this apparently inhibitory action in terms of Goldschmidt's theory of differential velocities in two concurrent developmental processes.

PLATE VII

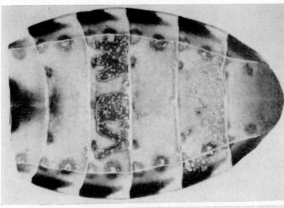

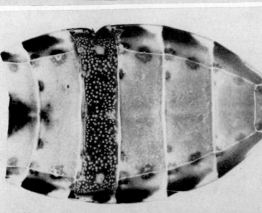

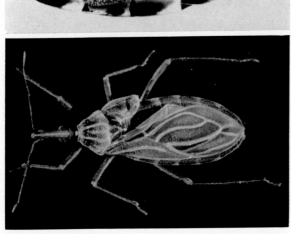

a, adult *Rhodnius* with a larval wing on the right side following the local application of juvenile hormone in the 5th-stage larva.

b, dorsal integument of the abdomen of an adult *Rhodnius* with one larval segment.

c, the same with initials marked out in larval cuticle on one segment.

In the moulting cycle of an insect there are two processes at work: (1) the exaggerated growth of certain parts of the epidermis, which leads to the changes in form of the ensuing instar, and (2) the deposition of the new cuticle, which terminates in the act of moulting.

Growth in the epidermis is possible only during the early phases of the moulting cycle, while the cells are detached from the cuticle. As soon as the deposition of a new cuticle begins, further growth is impossible. I therefore suggested that the corpus allatum hormone inhibits differentiation toward the adult form by accelerating those processes in the epidermal cell which lead to the deposition of the cuticle.

It was supposed (Fig. 33) that at each instar differentiation toward the adult begins, but is cut short by cuticle deposition before it has gone very far. At the final moult, however, when the corpus allatum hormone is absent, cuticle deposition is delayed and adult differentiation is completed.

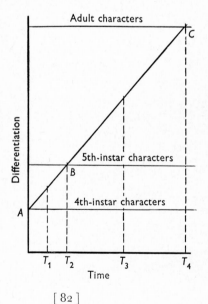

Fig. 33. Diagram to illustrate the earlier theory of control of metamorphosis in *Rhodnius*. Ordinate: differentiation of adult characters. Abscissa: time of deposition of new cuticle. In the moulting of a 4th-stage larva, if deposition of new cuticle occurred at T_1, characters would be intermediate between 4th and 5th instars; at T_2, 5th-instar characters appear; at T_3, characters are intermediate between 5th instar and adult; at T_4, adult characters appear.

This same idea is implicit in the writings of other authors. Thus Williams[114] has sometimes called the corpus allatum hormone the "status quo hormone"—implying, as the term "inhibitory hormone" did, that it inhibits adult differentiation.

There are many observations which fit in well with this interpretation. The moulting hormone is certainly secreted before the corpus allatum hormone. We have already seen how decapitation at the critical period, when the moulting hormone has been secreted, but before the corpus allatum hormone has been secreted, leads to precocious metamorphosis.

Fig. 34 represents a striking experiment.[100] If a 4th-stage larva A has another 4th-stage larva B joined to it, and both are at the same stage after feeding, A will develop into a nor-

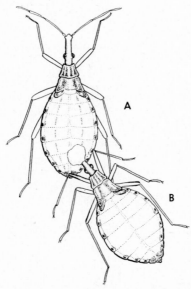

Fig. 34. Two 4th-stage larvae joined during different stages of the moulting process. Explanation in the text.

mal 5th-stage larva. But if A is at twenty-four hours after feeding, and B is at 7 days after feeding (so that it already contains corpus allatum hormone, and therefore A receives this hormone too early in the moulting process), differentiation toward the adult does not proceed so far as usual and characters develop in A which are intermediate between a 4th stage and a 5th stage.

Fig. 35 gives the results of another early experiment.[85] Fig. 35, A, shows the rudiments of the genitalia as seen in the 5th-instar larva of the male bedbug *Cimex*. The lateral appendages or claspers are asymmetrical, that on the left side being slightly larger. During the final moult the epidermal rudiments of both claspers develop for a time beneath the cuticle (Fig. 35, C), and then the right one atrophies and disappears and only the left one remains to form the hooklike clasper of the

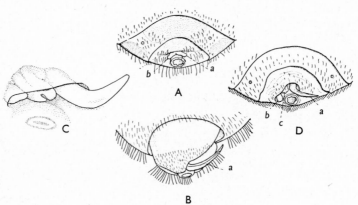

Fig. 35. Genital segments of male *Cimex,* ventral view, A, normal 5th-instar larva; B, normal adult; C, epidermal rudiments of the claspers, etc., in a male larva approaching the adult stage; D, a stage with characters intermediate between 5th instar and adult, produced by transfusing a decapitated 5th-instar larva with blood from a moulting 3rd-instar larva of *Rhodnius. a,* left clasper; *b,* right clasper; *c,* aedeagus.

adult male (Fig. 35, B). If graded doses of corpus allatum hormone from *Rhodnius* are given to the 5th-stage *Cimex*, a graded series of intermediates is obtained, with genitalia which reproduce exactly the intermediate stages shown by the epidermal rudiments (Fig. 35, D). It is difficult to avoid the impression that the corpus allatum hormone has caused these insects to lay down new cuticle precociously.

But when the growth processes during metamorphosis are studied closely, the hypothesis that this hormone merely inhibits differentiation toward the adult becomes untenable.

The most obvious change at metamorphosis is the exaggerated growth of special organs such as the wing lobes and genitalia. But there are specialized outgrowths also in the larva. The cuticle of the dorsum of the abdomen in the adult *Rhodnius* is relatively thin, with transverse folds and few bristles. The cuticle of the larva is a much more complex affair. The implantation of an active corpus allatum into the 5th-stage larva may lead to the production of an adult with a little patch of larval cuticle formed over the gland. Fig. 36 shows a section through such a preparation: the larval cuticle is far thicker and is adapted for stretching; the epicuticle is thrown into deep stellate folds, and the numerous innervated bristles are surrounded by smooth plaques (*cf*. Plate VIII, *b*).

In order to provide for the great distension of the abdomen which occurs at feeding, not only is the surface of the larval cuticle highly folded, but the number of epidermal cells per unit area is far greater than in the adult. In consequence, the histological changes during moulting are different from the outset, depending on whether a larval or an adult cuticle is to be formed. Whereas in the wing there is more active mitosis when metamorphosis occurs, in the abdomen there is far more active mitosis if a larval cuticle is to be laid down.

[85]

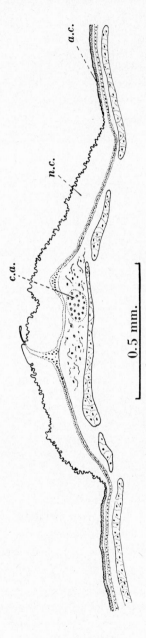

0.5 mm.

Fig. 36. Longitudinal section through a local patch of larval cuticle overlying an implanted corpus allatum in an adult *Rhodnius. c.a.,* implanted corpus allatum; *a.c.,* normal adult cuticle, thin with relatively thick exocuticle; *n.c.,* larval cuticle, very thick with highly folded epicuticle but no exocuticle. The epidermis below the larval cuticle has the nuclei more densely packed.

It is impossible to describe such differences as due to an inhibition of the outgrowth of adult structures. The corpus allatum hormone is clearly doing something active and positive in causing differentiated growth of larval type.

It was for this reason that since 1940[89] I have referred to this hormone as the juvenile hormone or (because I was urged to give it a Greek name) "neotenin," the youth substance— a substance which specifically evokes the formation of larval characters by the epidermis, when this is stimulated to grow under the action of the thoracic gland hormone "ecdyson."

This conclusion is reinforced by observations on the moulting of the adult insect. The adult *Rhodnius* can be induced to form a new cuticle if it is exposed experimentally to the moulting hormone, either by joining to it one or more moulting 5th-stage larvae (Fig. 37, A)[89] or by implanting an active thoracic gland.[99] The cuticle which it lays down is again of adult type (Plate VIII, *c*).

But if at the same time it is supplied with "juvenile hormone" by attaching a couple of 4th-stage larvae which retain

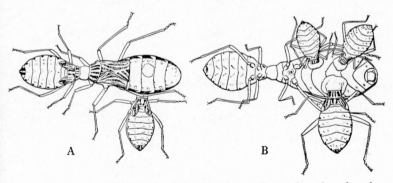

A   B

Fig. 37. A, adult *Rhodnius,* with wings cut short, decapitated and joined to two 5th-stage larvae; B, adult *Rhodnius,* decapitated and joined to two 5th-stage larvae and two 4th-stage larvae.

[87]

their corpora allata (Fig. 37, B), or by implanting a number of corpora allata from 3rd- or 4th-stage larvae, or by applying to the surface of the abdomen an active extract of juvenile hormone,[111] then the new cuticle over the surface of the abdomen shows a partial return to the larval type, with stellate folds and an attempt to form plaques (Plate VIII, *d*). In these insects, also, the number of epidermal cells per unit area is greatly increased beneath the regions of larval cuticle.

A partial reversal of metamorphosis of this kind cannot be described by a purely inhibitory action of the corpus allatum

PLATE VIII

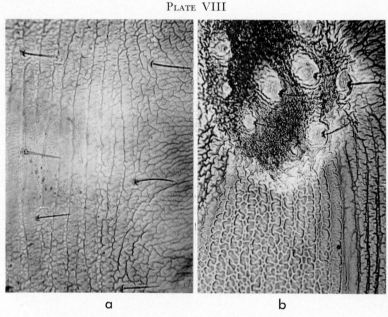

a   b

a, normal abdominal cuticle in adult *Rhodnius* with transverse folds and bristles without a surrounding area of smooth cuticle.

b, above, a patch of larval cuticle with stellate folding and bristles surrounded by smooth plaques; below, normal adult cuticle.

PLATE VIII—*Continued*

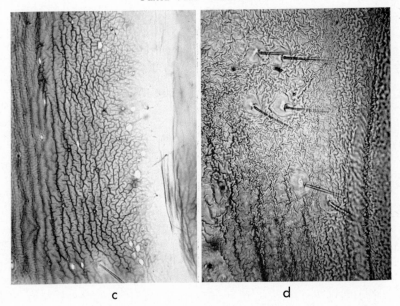

c   d

c, new cuticle formed when an adult was induced to moult in the absence of juvenile hormone; it is of normal adult type.

d, new cuticle formed when an adult was induced to moult in the presence of juvenile hormone; the stellate folding is of larval type, and the bristles are surrounded by smooth areas reminiscent of the plaques in the larva.

hormone. This hormone must be doing something more positive in evoking larval characters.

The discussion of that problem must be left until we have surveyed the general question of polymorphism in insects in the next chapter. Two further points may be added here. For anyone who has thought at all closely about insect metamorphosis in all its grades, slight and extreme, it is impossible not to be reminded of the metamorphosis that occurs in man at puberty. And those of us who have been working in this field have often speculated on whether there may not be a "juvenile hormone" in mammals.

It has long been known that precocious puberty in infants is associated with tumours of the adrenal. It is therefore exceedingly interesting that Gilbert and Schneiderman[24] should have succeeded in demonstrating the presence, in extracts of the suprarenal cortex of the ox, of a substance, apparently a steroid, which shows juvenile hormone activity when injected into insects; and Williams et al.[117] have found that this substance is widely distributed in mammalian tissues. Whether it is indeed playing a comparable role in the mammal remains to be seen.

The other point we may consider here concerns the evolution of the control of "metamorphosis" by the corpus allatum.

It has been shown by M. J. Wells[81] that in the *Octopus* a glandular organ behind the brain has the function of inhibiting the development of the gonads until the animal is fully grown. Some regulation of this kind is clearly necessary in any bisexual animal; and this is perhaps the starting point for the evolution of the hormonal control of metamorphosis.

Thus we may picture an animal (with its gonad development inhibited) evolving a larval form adapted to the particular conditions of its growth. The inhibition of gonad development is then removed, and the maturation of the gonads coincides with the disappearance of the larval form. According to this idea, which has been developed by Wells, the control of metamorphosis by the corpus allatum may be considered a secondary effect, the primary step being the control of gonad development.

v · Polymorphism

THE subject of growth and form becomes increasingly difficult as the argument proceeds. In the last chapter we discussed the evidence for the view that the epidermal cells throughout the body of the young *Rhodnius* have dual potentialities. In the growing insect one of these potentialities, that of the larval form, is manifest; the other, that of the adult form, is latent within the cells. But, nonetheless, this latent adult form, which cannot be seen, exists in a pattern over the surface of the body which is as well defined as the visible form of the larva.

The realization of these two forms is controlled by the timing and concentration of the secretion of juvenile hormone by the corpus allatum. Too high a concentration of juvenile hormone or the supply of this hormone too early in the moulting process causes undue suppression of the emergence of adult characters, and the larval form is retained. When young larvae are caused to moult in the absence of the juvenile hormone, the adult characters appear.

Disturbances in the normal balance of these two hormones lead to abnormalities in metamorphosis: the condition known as prothetely, the precocious appearance of adult characters in larvae, or that called metathetely, the retention of larval characters in the adult stage. Silkworms with antennae were recorded more than a century and a half ago; and this abnormality has been produced experimentally by Fukuda[23] by implanting an active prothoracic gland into a 5th-stage larva early in the instar, at a time when a little juvenile hormone secretion is still occurring. Such disturbances may result from abnormal temperatures, which influence one hormone more than the other; or they may commonly arise in species hybrids in which the normal hormone balance has become deranged.[84]

When elaborate structures such as the wings are to be fully differentiated, a certain minimum number of cells is necessary. If the 1st-stage larva of *Rhodnius* is caused to moult directly to an adult by decapitating it and attaching it to the tip of the head of a moulting 5th-stage larva, the tiny lobes on the thorax give rise to little crumpled membranes which are a very poor imitation of wings (Fig. 38). So few cells are present that they are not yet "competent" to develop into proper wings; but that does not affect the general principle.

In order to avoid obscuring the argument with a host of special instances, the discussion in this book has been confined almost entirely to the epidermis of *Rhodnius*. But at this point it will be well to say a word or two about metamorphosis in holometabolous insects in which a pupal stage intervenes between the larva and the adult.

The principles of control are here the same, but we have an organism with three potential variants, the larva, the pupa, and the imago or adult. As was first shown by Bounhiol,[8] if the corpora allata in a young caterpillar are extirpated, it turns directly into a pupa at the next moult, and this gives rise to a diminutive adult (Fig. 39). It is therefore sometimes said that the formation of the pupa marks the real point at which meta-

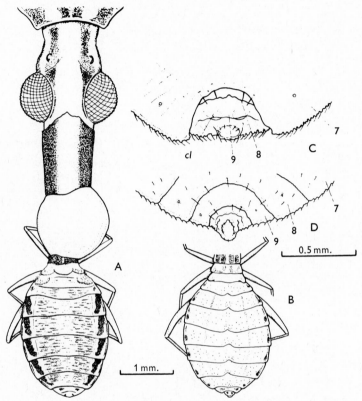

Fig. 38. A, precocious adult produced from 1st-stage larva by joining it to head of a moulting 5th-stage larva. B, normal 2nd-stage larva for comparison; C, terminal segments of the precocious (male); D, the same in normal 2nd-stage larva. The numbers indicate homologous segments; *cl,* claspers.

morphosis occurs and that the pupa is perhaps to be regarded as a first adult instar.

However that may be, the physiological principle seems to be the same as in *Rhodnius:* the three forms are controlled by the timing and concentration of juvenile hormone secretion. The larva is formed in the presence of much juvenile hormone,

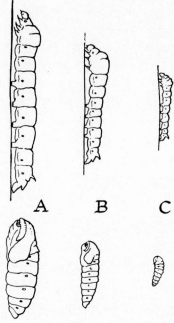

Fig. 39. Precocious metamorphosis in the silkworm. (After Bounhiol.) A, above, larva 7 days after final moult; below, the pupa resulting from starvation of such a larva. B, above, larva 4–5 days after third moult; below, pupa resulting from ablation of corpora allata at this stage. C, above, larva 3–4 days after second moult; below, pupa after ablation of corpora allata.

the pupa when only a very little is present, the adult when the hormone is absent.

If the corpus allatum of the last-stage larva of the bee is eliminated by ligaturing off the head, so that the juvenile hormone is abnormally reduced in amount, the resulting pupa shows characters which are intermediate between those of a normal pupa and an adult bee.[70] The same happens in *Hyalophora* when the corpus allatum is removed in the last larval stage.[116] And it was shown by Nayar,[48] working in my laboratory, that if a piece of larval cuticle of the wax moth *Galleria* is implanted into the integument of a pupa it will give rise to a patch of integument bearing structures which are clearly rudimentary scales: the stage with pupal cuticle has been partially suppressed.

The partial reversal of metamorphosis which was discussed in the preceding chapter is of great theoretical significance in this connection; and it is fortunate that the same phenomenon has been described in Lepidoptera by Piepho.[53,54] If a cylindrical segment of the head or of a limb in *Rhodnius* is implanted into the abdomen, the epidermis will grow outward to unite with itself and thus forms a closed capsule which will then proceed to moult simultaneously with its host.[85] This technique was later used extensively by Piepho in *Galleria*, and he showed that pupal cuticle implanted in a young larva will moult to give larval cuticle again (though sometimes several moults are necessary before reversal comes about); occasionally even adult cuticle can be caused to revert to pupal and to larval cuticle and then go forward again to lay down adult cuticle with scales.[57,82]

All these results serve to emphasize that metamorphosis is not to be thought of as a progressive "differentiation" of adult characters. It is rather to be regarded as the successive realization of alternative latent forms.

When alternative forms normally succeed one another in the course of the life cycle of a single animal, the phenomenon was termed by Lubbock[44] "polyeidism," in order to distinguish it from what is commonly called "polymorphism," in which a given individual of the species assumes either one form or another. But the two phenomena have so much in common that it is instructive to think of them together; and the purpose of this chapter is to consider some of the examples of poly-

morphism in insects with a view to comparing them with metamorphosis.

For many people the most familiar type of polymorphism
within a species is that brought about by mutant genes. Great
numbers of such mutant forms of *Drosophila* are maintained
in the sheltered conditions of the laboratory; and it is not un-
common to find such mutants existing in nature. Among
Lepidoptera, for example, E. B. Ford[20] recognizes two types
of genetic polymorphism. In one type, termed by him "bal-
anced polymorphism," the different forms, often strikingly dis-
similar in appearance, exist side by side. That is seen, for example, among mimetic butterflies, when different forms of the
female mimic a series of widely different species. The characters of the polymorphic mimics are controlled by a rather
complex system of interacting genes, and the various forms
occur in more or less constant proportions.

The other type of polymorphism is termed by Ford "transi-
ent polymorphism." The classic example is the melanism that
has appeared during the past century in many different species
of Lepidoptera in the industrial areas of Europe. Here again
both forms exist side by side, but there is good experimental
evidence to show that the black mutant is being progressively
favoured by natural selection in those areas where the lichens
have been eliminated and the tree trunks blackened by the
pollution of the atmosphere.

In these examples the relative numbers of the different
forms that appear in the offspring during breeding experiments
conform well enough to the classic laws of Mendel. But there
are other examples of genetic polymorphism in which these
laws do not hold, because the "penetrance" of the gene or the
manifestation of the mutant character is greatly influenced by

the environment. It is this type of polymorphism which is particularly instructive from our present point of view.

Under the action of the *tetraptera* gene in *Drosophila* the little knobbed halteres are changed to wings. But this effect is greatly influenced by temperature: at 25°C. the "penetrance" of *tetraptera* is 35 per cent, at 17°C. it is only 1 per cent.[3] In *tetraltera*, in which the wings are changed to halteres, there is a converse effect: at 29°C. the penetrance is only 1 per cent, at 14°C. 35 per cent; and food which leads to a prolongation of development will likewise increase the penetrance of *tetraltera*.[76]

Similarly in *aristopedia,* in which the arista of the antenna in *Drosophila* becomes more or less leglike, cold treatment (14.5°C.) increases the expression, and heat treatment (29°C.) decreases it.[76] In *proboscipedia,* in which the oral lobes of the proboscis may come to resemble labrum, maxillary palps, antennae, or tarsi, changes in temperature may suppress the effect and lead to the formation of normal mouth parts.[9] In general, in this mutant, cold treatment (15°C.) favours the appearance of aristalike appendages on the proboscis, heat treatment (29°C.) results in the development of tarsuslike appendages.[77]

It can even happen that the same abnormalities may appear in normal strains of *Drosophila* when these are subjected to some unusual temperature shock or other adverse stimulus at the appropriate "sensitive" period of growth. For example, if the *Drosophila* egg is exposed to a temperature shock[46] or to ether vapour[25,31] during a period of 15 minutes at 3 hours after fertilization, a large proportion of the resulting flies have the metathorax more or less completely changed into a mesothorax, exactly as is brought about by the gene "bithorax."[46]

I do not intend to discuss at length just how these various

[97]

stimuli are bringing about these striking morphological differences. Many authors, and notably Goldschmidt, have thought in terms of chemical evocators, specific for the various structures, diffusing into the organ rudiment at some critical moment of development and thus leading to the formation of a given type of organ, or of evocators produced within the nucleus of every cell in an imaginal disc, which can exert their determining influence only when the cell has reached the right state of competence.[77]

The point that I want to emphasize is that the capacity to form these different types of appendage is latent within the cells of the imaginal disc, just as the capacity to form innervated bristles, dermal glands, oenocytes, or ordinary cuticle is latent within the epidermal cells of the *Rhodnius* abdomen; or as the capacity to form larval, pupal, or imaginal cuticle resides within the same cells in Lepidoptera.

The stimuli which provoke these changes in *aristopedia* and the other mutants that we have been considering—such things as temperature, general nutrition, and narcotics—are of a somewhat indefinite nature: the immediate cause of the observed changes is not known. But there are other morphological mutants in which more exact knowledge is available.

If *Drosophila* larvae of the mutant *antennaless,* in which the antennae usually fail to appear, are given a diet rich in riboflavine, they will develop normal antennae.[28] Kynurenine or its oxidation products will lead to normal eye coloration if supplied to the *vermilion* mutant (*v*) of *Drosophila* or the red-eyed mutant (*a*) of *Ephestia*.[19] Various iminazol derivatives and, indeed, many other substances have a so-called "antibar" effect and cause the development of normal eyes when administered to *bar* eye mutants of *Drosophila* in which the number of facets would otherwise be greatly reduced.[13, 15]

In these examples the manifestation of the mutant condition has been suppressed by a specific chemical substance. These effects may not be precisely comparable with the action of inductors, but they do serve to show the striking and specific morphological changes that can be brought about by the presence or absence of a single chemical.

We can approach the problem of polymorphism in insects from another angle, by observing the more general effects of environment on morphology. Here, again, the environment is presumably controlling, in some way or other, the functioning of the various genes.

Sex in insects as in other animals is genetically determined; that is, the latent capacity to form male or female parts is controlled by the balance of male and female determinants in the sex chromosomes and autosomes which have been brought together at fertilization. But this genetic balance can be upset. In the classic work of Goldschmidt[26, 27] on intersexes in the gipsy moth *Lymantria,* it is upset by a disturbance in the relative "strength" of the male and female determinants when different races are crossed. In the extreme cases, insects with the genetic constitution of one sex may be normally functioning individuals of the opposite sex.

Sex characters may also be upset by nutrition. If the tissues of various Hymenoptera are deprived of nourishment by the presence of internal parasites (notably *Stylops*), there is often a partial suppression of the genetic sex and the appearance of the characters of the opposite sex.[64, 65] Presumably the defective nutrition of the cells, perhaps in respect to some specific substance, has changed the balance of sex determiners within them.

Other characters may be similarly influenced by nutrition. Schmieder[72] has described how the ichneumonid *Melittobia,* which develops within the body of other Hymenoptera, is strikingly affected. These ichneumonid parasites are poly-embryonic: a single egg fragments during development in the host to produce some hundreds of embryos. When *Melittobia* develops in a host large enough to provide sustenance for 500–800 larvae, the first twenty or so to develop are brachypterous (short-winged) females and eyeless males. All the remainder, receiving perhaps different food, develop into adults of normal form.

Males of the minute chalcid *Trichogramma semblidis* are apterous when reared from the eggs of *Sialis,* but winged and with striking differences in the morphology of the legs and antennae when reared from the eggs of *Ephestia* and other Lepidoptera (Fig. 40).[66, 67] Perhaps the dimorphism in the agamic and gamic generations of female cynipids (the gall wasps) is due to their developing in different parts of the host plant.[68]

In the ichneumonid *Gelis,* the female is always wingless, but the male is fully winged if it is fed adequately in the larval stage. On the other hand, if the male larvae are reared throughout in a small host or are removed from a large host before they have finished feeding, they develop into mi-

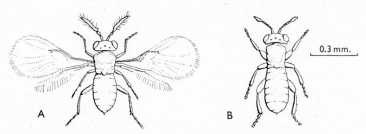

Fig. 40. Dimorphism in the male of *Trichogramma semblidis.* (After Salt.) A, winged male reared in egg of Lepidoptera; B, apterous male reared in egg of *Sialis.*

cropterous males which differ from the normal not only in the development of the wings, but in the structure of the thorax, the size of the ocelli, the form of the endoskeleton, and the development, innervation, and tracheal supply of the thoracic muscles; and there are no intermediates.[69]

In all these examples, some nutritional change, which perhaps means a change in the supply of some single chemical substance, has led to an abrupt change in form in many different parts of the body. The whole phenomenon has much in common with the effects of the juvenile hormone in controlling metamorphosis. The epidermal cells of *Rhodnius* contain within them the gene complex and the potential enzymes capable of producing either larval or adult structures. It is the selective activation of this system in the presence or absence of the juvenile hormone which controls the form of the body.

In the present state of knowledge it is impossible to say just how a simple chemical substance leads to the activation of one set of genes or of enzymes to the exclusion of another set. Hormones seem often to be token stimulators. They are, as it were, keys which will open particular doors; what is inside these doors bears no relation to the properties of the key.

Besides the control of metamorphosis the juvenile hormone will control the deposition of yolk in the eggs—and doubtless other metabolic functions. It may well play a part in some of the other polymorphisms that occur in insects.

In grasshoppers or locusts there are often two "phases" (which at one time were regarded as separate species), a gregarious phase which builds up into destructive swarms and a solitary phase which is a harmless creature. There is evidence that some, at least, of the characters of the solitary phase can be produced by the implantation of corpora allata; and Kennedy[37] has suggested that the solitary phase may perhaps be regarded as a slightly juvenile form, a neotenic form of the species. This idea is supported by the fact that some other Orthoptera are certainly neotenic in some degree. The stick insect *Dixippus* never acquires the full adult characters seen in other stick insects, but starts to reproduce when the outward characters are more or less immature. Even the adult cockroach must be slightly larval in form, for if the corpora allata are removed from a cockroach before the final moult, the resulting adult shows a greater degree of metamorphosis than usual; it becomes a kind of "superadult."[6]

The termites are another group of insects which show a remarkable degree of polymorphism. Here again there is evidence that the juvenile hormone may be involved, for the implantation of extra corpora allata into termite larvae leads to the production of "soldiers," forms with powerful mandibles, which may perhaps be regarded as "superlarvae," extra juvenile forms.[45]

In the developing larva of an insect, all the cells have dual or triple potentialities. Which of these potentialities is realized, which system of enzymes becomes functional, is determined by the presence or absence of what must be a comparatively simple chemical substance, the juvenile hormone. According to the view that is here put forward, the larva, pupa, and adult of an insect represent different forms in a polymorphic organism, the realization of which is controlled by the timing and the amount of the juvenile hormone secretion.

The manifestation of these forms is dependent on the synthetic activity of the epidermal cells. The juvenile hormone must be reacting with the gene-controlled enzyme system of these cells in such a way as to deflect morphogenesis by its influence on particular syntheses. Cells activated by the moulting hormone alone develop their adult characters; if a small amount of juvenile hormone is present, pupal characters appear; and if a large amount of juvenile hormone is present, larval characters are developed (Fig. 41).

The nature of the action of the moulting hormone has already been considered; I suggested that it facilitates in some way the access to their substrates of the enzymes concerned in protein synthesis. As regards the juvenile hormone, I have been inclined in the past to think of this as some kind of a coenzyme, which favours the activity of those enzymes concerned in the realization of larval characters. But it is possible to conceive that it, also, is concerned in the regulation of permeability relations within the cells, in such a way that the gene-controlled enzyme system which is responsible for larval characters is brought increasingly into action when the juvenile hormone

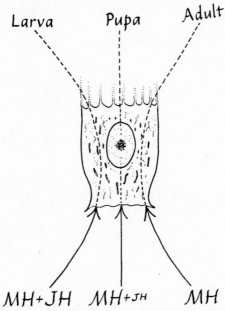

Fig. 41. Hormonal control of metamorphosis in epidermal cell acted upon by moulting hormone (*M.H.*) and juvenile hormone (*J.H.*) in different proportions.

is present. Or we can say that the juvenile hormone is activating those genes that are concerned in larval syntheses.

The objection has been made that it is of little help in the understanding of metamorphosis to try to explain this by reference to another phenomenon, polymorphism, which is itself not understood. The answer is that metamorphosis viewed in this light is no longer a unique phenomenon, but only a particularly striking manifestation of a property that is universal in living organisms. That means that the study of metamorphosis may throw light upon other, more general, phenomena of growth.

Metamorphosis is an example of highly divergent forms of the body being produced in genetically uniform material. The other familiar example of diversity appearing between cells which may be presumed to have uniform genetic constitutions is the difference in form of the different parts of the body.

When discussing the differentiation of the epidermal cells in *Rhodnius* into dermal glands and bristle-forming centres and their components (p. 29), I put forward the view that the control of such differentiation might lie in the supply or deficiency of specific raw materials. These hypothetical materials were thought of as being produced locally within the tissues and absorbed by one part in preference to another. Substances of this kind are termed "inductors," and they result in autonomous differentiation of the tissues.

That conception has much in common with the polymorphism of whole organisms that we have been discussing in this chapter and with the control of metamorphosis by the supply or deficiency of the juvenile hormone. The only essential difference is that the juvenile hormone is not produced locally within the tissues but is the product of an endocrine gland and is circulating as a hormone in the tissue fluids.

VI · The Integration
of Growth

IN the preceding chapters we have come some way toward describing the endocrine control of the activities of the epidermal cell. We must now consider how this control is integrated to ensure the co-ordinated growth of the whole animal. In the present state of knowledge it is impossible to formulate a theory of the integration of growth that is sharply defined. The questions to be considered are difficult and the present answers are obscure; but it is worth while considering these questions if only in the hope that we shall thereby be able to formulate them more clearly.

As the body grows, many of the cells die and undergo autolysis; and the integration of this process of cell death may be as important as that of cell multiplication. It is seen at its simplest in the epidermis. During the height of cell division in the epidermis of *Rhodnius* and other insects[90,95] mitosis is so exuberant that many more cells are produced than will be needed to form the new integument. The unwanted cells die; the nucleus disintegrates to form a number of Feulgen-positive "chromatin droplets" which are apparently assimilated by the neighboring cells; and gradually, as mitosis comes to an end, a regular sheet of epidermal cells is formed in which the nuclei are evenly spaced (Fig. 42). The deposition of the new cuticle can now begin.

When the *Rhodnius* larva undergoes metamorphosis to the adult, the number of bristles on the cuticle of the abdomen is greatly reduced. The bristle- and socket-forming cells therefore disappear during the final moult. They undergo "histolysis" in just the same way as the unwanted cells produced by excessive cell division.

Another example of histolysis, already mentioned, is that which affects the thoracic gland when the insect becomes adult (Fig. 22). This has been studied experimentally in *Rhodnius* in some detail.[104]

If the gland is removed from a newly moulted adult (say within half an hour of moulting), it will break down in any

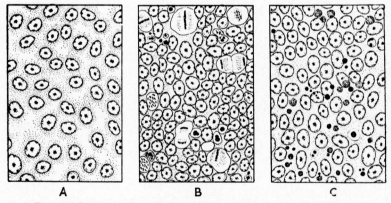

A   B   C

Fig. 42. Corresponding regions of the epidermis of the abdomen in *Rhodnius* 5th-stage larva, seen in surface view at different times after feeding. A, 3 days, cell division not begun; B, 8 days, active mitosis, cells densely packed, nuclear breakdown beginning; C, 13 days, cells less dense, abundant chromatin droplets resulting from breakdown of excess nuclei.

[106]

environment. Even if it is transplanted into a young larval stage containing juvenile hormone, its autolysis cannot be prevented: its breakdown is already "determined," although, in outward appearance, the cells look entirely healthy.

But if the gland is taken out a day or two before moulting to the adult, it behaves quite differently: it will not break down even when transplanted into a newly moulted adult. And the gland taken from a newly moulted 5th-stage larva likewise will not break down when transplanted to a newly moulted adult or, indeed, to any other stage.

From such experiments we must conclude that two factors are concerned in bringing about histolysis of the thoracic gland.

First, at the time of moulting to the adult the gland receives a humoral stimulus (factor A) which leads to its breakdown; and after exposure to this stimulus it will break down in any environment. It cannot be saved, for example, by transplanting to an insect with active juvenile hormone.

Second, this stimulus to autolysis (factor A) is effective only if the gland has come from a 5th-stage larva which is moulting to an adult; that is, if the gland has passed through a moulting cycle in the absence of the juvenile hormone. Exposure of the gland to the juvenile hormone causes no visible change in the cells, but it affects them in some way so that they no longer break down when exposed to factor A.

We do not know what effect the juvenile hormone is exerting upon the cells, which prevents their subsequent histolysis. All we can say is that these cells have retained their larval properties and therefore do not break down when exposed to factor A.

Nor do we know the nature or the source of factor A. This is certainly a hormonal stimulus of some kind; for the thoracic gland in *Rhodnius* receives no nerve supply, and the gland is influenced in just the same way, and caused to undergo histolysis shortly after moulting, even when it has been transplanted to another part of the body.

The histolysis of the thoracic gland happens to have been studied experimentally and has therefore been described at some length. But it is merely one example of a widespread phenomenon—the dissolution at metamorphosis of all those structures characteristic of the larva, which is so striking in holometabolous insects. This process does not differ in principle from the more limited histolysis in the epidermis of *Rhodnius*. It occurs chiefly in the pupal stage; but some breakdown continues in the adult after moulting. In such flies as *Musca* or *Drosophila* the larval fat body is still intact in the young adult; it disappears during the next few days just like the thoracic gland.[98]

This process of selective cell death is just one aspect of the integration of growth. The main problem we have to consider is how the body grows as a whole. Here we can recognize three mechanisms of co-ordination:

(1) Direct physical contact and continuity from one cell to the next.

(2) The transmission of stimuli by nerves from the periphery to the central nervous system, leading to the central control of growth.

(3) The distribution of chemical messengers (hormones) by the blood stream throughout the body, which ensures the simultaneous growth of all its parts.

The continuity or contact between the individual epidermal cells is of the first importance. That is well seen during wound healing. No matter how sparse and attenuated the epidermal cells become as the result of migration to a wound, they never let go of one another (Fig. 15). And wound healing comes to an end when continuity is again restored in the epidermal sheet of cells. The same continuity must play an essential part in the gradients which undoubtedly exist in the epidermis.

What is the nature of this continuity? At the present time we can do no more than speculate. I like to picture some specific interaction between the cell substance of the cells in contact, something, perhaps, in the nature of an antigen-antibody reaction which would result in the specific binding of the cells together by physical and chemical bonds of varying degrees of strength.

The epidermal cells which are pictured as being bound together in this way possess, as we have seen, some kind of cytoskeleton which confers a permanent orientation or polarity on the cell. If the epidermal cell has such an organized protein framework which is chemically linked to the framework of the adjacent cells, then, without too great a strain on the meaning of words, we can regard the whole assembly as a chemical continuum, comparable with a highly heterogeneous plastic.

It is in this sense that I (in common with such distinguished predecessors as Edouard Pflüger) have suggested that the living organism is to be thought of as a "giant molecule." [92, 96] No such continuity exists between the free and independent amoeboid cells of *Acrasia*. But when they come together and combine to form the fruiting body, we are witnessing the formation of such a continuum, a continuum which is the necessary condition for morphological development.

The alternative is to regard all the parts as independent and as influencing one another from a distance by the exchange of chemical messages or in some other way. There is no doubt that such exchanges are taking place. Indeed, a specific chemical substance "acrasin" provokes the aggregation of the migrating amoeboid forms of *Acrasia*. The existence of hor-

mones is the clearest example; and there is increasing evidence
that the different organs can communicate by the production
of organ-specific products. But such chemical messengers are
operating in a system whose main framework has already
been established by other means.

This way of looking at the organism as a chemical continuum has the advantage of being equally applicable to cellular and noncellular forms. The insect begins life as a noncellular organism. The egg is a single cell (Fig. 43). At a
certain stage of development (there are differences in different

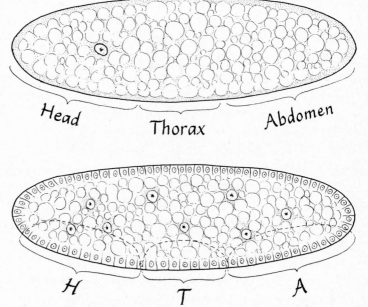

Fig. 43. Above, insect egg at time of laying, with single nucleus
(germinal vesicle) in the yolk. The prospective regions of the germ
band zone are indicated. Below, the same after the completion of
cleavage and formation of the blastoderm. The yolk contains vitello-
phags.

insects, but the principle applies throughout) the "organism" consists of an apparently uniform sheet of cytoplasm in the cortex of the oocyte. This sheet contains no nuclei and no cell walls, but (in some insects at least, such as *Drosophila* or the housefly) its different parts are already "determined" to form different parts of the insect.

To my mind, almost the only possible way of thinking about this "organism" is to regard it as an inconceivably complex continuum of protein chains, which compose and support the enzyme systems that characterize the various parts.

The cortical plasma in the germ band region of the egg differentiates to form the embryo. If it is split lengthways with a needle, it will form two embryos. Its parts must therefore contain all the materials which, in the presence of the egg nucleus and, of course, the reserves in the yolk, is capable of producing a complete organism.

It is this material which is thought of as a "lipid-nucleoprotein-plastic" or "macromolecule," the parts of which can be differently activated or modified to set in motion the sequence of changes that lead ultimately to differences in enzyme content and so to visible differences in growth in the various parts.

The idea which is difficult to grasp is that of a substrate sufficiently complex to differentiate into a complete embryo and yet sufficiently homogeneous for it to be capable of being divided to form two embryos.

Perhaps the key to this paradox is to be found in the interaction between cytoplasm and nucleus. We may imagine a series of reactive sites in the nucleoprotein plastic of the cytoplasm, each of which is subject to the action of the series of genes in the nucleus. The initial reaction will occur at the most favoured site. This site is favoured because the concentration of some essential reactant (oxygen, for example) is greater there.

That is the well-known conception of "gradients" which has been so extensively developed by C. M. Child.

Whatever may be the mechanism of the process, it has been abundantly proved that when one site in a system of this kind becomes activated for a particular line of development the surrounding sites are prevented from undergoing the same change. But secondary modifications can now take place, again by the interaction between favoured sites in the cytoplasm and the genes in the nucleus; and these altered centres again prevent the surrounding sites from undergoing the same change. The possible mechanisms of this process were discussed in Chapter II.

We now have the rudiments of an organism. It is still perhaps a continuum of "lipid-nucleoprotein" reticular chains, but particular parts are the formative centres of enzyme systems which, as they become active, provide the basis for the appearance of structural differences.

A unicellular protozoan is presumably a system of this kind. And it is helpful to find in the protozoa an example of a cell component which is capable of giving rise to a differentiated whole even though subdivided. Such an example is provided by the macronucleus. The protozoan macronucleus appears to be highly polyploid and contains, scattered through all its parts, all the genes necessary for development. Small fragments of cytoplasm from an organism such as *Stentor* will regenerate completely provided they contain a portion of the macronucleus.

The alternative to this picture of the organism, at the outset of its development, as a chemical continuum is to think of the noncellular rudiment of the organism as made up of independent parts which maintain their mutual relations and react upon one another by means of forces acting at a distance.

For me a discontinuous system of that kind is an almost impossibly difficult conception. We are familiar, of course, with organized societies of men or animals. But these are linked together by the controlling activities of an elaborate nervous system and organs of communication that are within each member of the community. When the unit in the community is an unattached group of enzymes at a point in the plasma, it is difficult to conceive a co-ordination of that kind. I find it necessary to picture some sort of continuity; hence the conception of a chemical continuity, as in a high polymer or plastic.

What I have been trying to outline is a conception of the organism, at the outset of its development, which can be described in physical and chemical terms. It is no more than a hypothesis, a way of thinking about the organization of living matter. But, as differentiation and growth proceed, physiological methods of integration and control, which are amenable to experimental study, come into existence.

The cleavage nuclei make their way to the surface of the egg, and those of them which happen to fall within the germ band zone become the antecedents of the embryo (Fig. 43). Their descendants become the epidermal cells which are the object of our study. I myself believe that a "cytoskeleton" still exists within the epidermal cell, that this framework is held continuous with the framework of neighboring cells, and that the resulting general framework remains the basis of the unity of the body. But, for the present, that is a hypothesis beyond the range of experiment. On the experimental plane we are concerned only with the more obvious forms of integration which develop as growth proceeds.

Certain cells within the epidermis become differentiated to form sense cells from which axon processes grow inward and finally become intimately associated with one another in the neuropile of the central nervous system (Fig. 44). Throughout their course these axons are insulated from neighboring axons by their neurilemmal sheaths. It is only in the synapses of the central neuropile that these special ectoderm cells come into intimate contact with one another.

I do not think that it is too far-fetched to liken this synaptic association of the sensory neurones to the intimate association of the peripheral epidermal cells with one another. However that may be, it clearly provides for the establishment of contacts between widely scattered regions of the epidermis. That is the basis of the sensory side of the central nervous system.

Other ectodermal cells make their way into the central nervous system to form association neurones which link the sensory neurones to the effector system. All these structures are specialized derivatives of the epidermis. We have already pointed out (p. 32) that well into postembryonic development new sensory neurones can arise and grow inward: the capacity to form the sensory side of the central nervous system still remains latent within the ordinary epidermal cell.

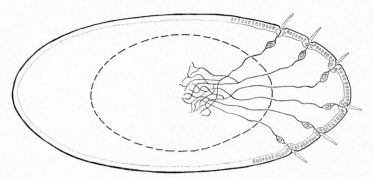

Fig. 44. Schematic figure showing the endings in the central nervous system of the neurones from the dermal sense organs.

Meanwhile, other local specializations have been taking place in the epidermis. Groups of epidermal cells in the region of the mouth parts multiply to form nests of cells which become detached and move inward to form the glands of internal secretion: the corpus allatum and the thoracic gland (Fig. 45).

The final link is provided by the effector neurones in the central nervous system. These also are specialized ectodermal cells which have migrated inward and link the neuropile of the sensory axons with the effector organs: the muscles and the glands—including the corpus allatum and, in some insects, the thoracic gland.

The last components to be mentioned are the neurosecretory cells in the central nervous system. The phylogenetic origin of these is still uncertain, but it has been suggested by Hanström [34, 35] that they may have been originally glands of ectodermal origin which have later become enclosed within the central

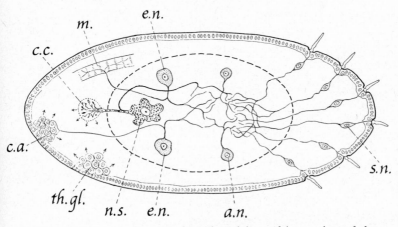

Fig. 45. Schematic figure to show the origins and interactions of the neuroendocrine system in an insect. *a.n.,* association neurone; *c.a.,* corpus allatum; *c.c.,* corpus cardiacum; *e.n.,* effector neurone; *m.,* muscle; *n.s.,* neurosecretory cell; *s.n.,* sensory neurone; *th.gl.,* thoracic gland.

nervous system. When we consider how close is the relationship between sensilla and dermal glands, even in *Rhodnius,* that is not an improbable suggestion.

The neurosecretory cells with which we are concerned come to lie in the dorsum of the pars intercerebralis of the proto-cerebrum. Their axons run to the corpus cardiacum. The secretion produced in the large bodies of these cells passes down the axons and accumulates in their swollen extremities in the corpus cardiacum, whence it is discharged into the cir-culating blood.

The purpose of this schematic picture of insect embryology is to emphasize that all these elements are products of the ectoderm and they are merely displaying in exaggerated form the properties that are already present in the ordinary epider-mal cells: the property of conduction of stimuli through points of contact with one another, the property of secretion of active substances, and the property of movement.

How far can we claim to understand the integration of growth on the basis of this system?

We know that the *Rhodnius* larva is caused to renew its growth when the abdomen is distended by a large meal. Such distension provides a nervous stimulus to the brain; if the nervous connection is severed by cutting the nerve cord in the neck, growth and moulting fail to occur.[84] This stimulus acti-vates the neurosecretory cells and sets in motion the sequence of humoral secretions which initiate growth in all parts of the body. But adequate nutrition is also necessary: larvae which imbibe lymph alone fail to moult. Clearly, the composition of the haemolymph is important.

There are other factors which may arrest the normal process of growth after a full meal. It is not surprising that the process is greatly prolonged by low temperature. But it is adversely affected by high temperature also. The speed of growth and moulting in *Rhodnius* reaches an optimum at about 30°C. If the temperature is raised still further, the interval between feeding and moulting is prolonged (Fig. 46). At 34°C. some 10 per cent of larvae fail to moult altogether. At 35°C., 50 per cent fail; and at 36°C. none moult.[100] Yet digestion and excretion and all the other physiological activities of these larvae proceed normally. The lethal temperature (the temperature at which 50 per cent of larvae are killed by an exposure of twenty-four hours) is about 40°C.

This adverse effect of moderately high temperature may well be exerted in part upon the brain and the neurosecretory cells. (The thoracic gland shows no histological signs of activation at 36°C.) But the effect is far more general than that; for decapitated larvae injected with abundant ecdyson also fail to moult at 36°C.[105] This high temperature is interfering with the action of the hormone on the epidermal cells.

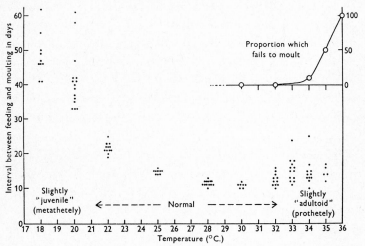

Fig. 46. Effect of temperature on the moulting of 4th-stage larvae of *Rhodnius.*

Growth can also be arrested by injury from extensive wounds or burns. It is clearly in the interests of the animal that that should be so; but it is not easy to see how uninjured parts of the body are informed, so that the steps leading to moulting shall not proceed.

One of the tissues which is always involved in injury is the haemolymph. This contains large numbers of free blood cells or haemocytes which collect around the wound, phagocytosing the dying cells and walling off the site.[86] By injecting substances such as Indian ink or iron saccharate through a fine capillary inserted into one of the appendages, it is easy to involve practically all the phagocytic haemocytes in the body in this activity, and they quickly become laden with debris; yet so little damage to the other tissues is produced that this injury by itself will have no effect on growth.

When injection is done during the first few days of the moulting cycle, that is, before the critical period, growth is completely arrested for several weeks (Fig. 47). On the fourth day after feeding, that is, after the critical period, such injections have no effect.[105]

This treatment does not interfere with the activity of the thoracic gland hormone; for if ecdyson is injected at the same time as the Indian ink, the haemocytes are blocked as usual but growth and moulting proceed at the normal rate.

In an attempt to explain these results several possibilities were considered: (1) that the haemocytes might be concerned in the production and secretion of some metabolic product necessary for the activation of the thoracic gland; (2) that these cells might be needed in order to transport the brain hormone from the corpus cardiacum to the thoracic gland; (3) that in the course of their phagocytic activity the haemocytes remove from the blood the hormone secreted by the brain.

None of these suggestions is proved; the actual mechanism of integration is unknown.

But, alongside these observations on the haemocytes, it is interesting to consider the results obtained by O'Farrell and Stock[50] on the regeneration of limbs in the cockroach. If a limb is removed from a young cockroach, a new limb may be regenerated during moulting. But the degree of regeneration depends on the time at which the injury is suffered.

If the leg is removed well before the next moult is due, this moult is delayed, perhaps for several weeks; and when it does occur, a completely normal leg has been regenerated. But if the leg is removed only a short time before the next moult is

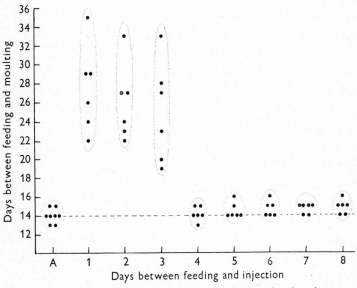

Fig. 47. Effect of blockage of the haemocytes on the time between feeding and moulting in the 4th-stage larva of *Rhodnius*. An injection of 5 mm.³ of 2 per cent iron saccharate was made into batches of six larvae on the first to the eighth day after feeding. A, control batch of eight which received no injection.

due, there is no delay at all in moulting, and only a small papilla is developed at the site of the injury. The useful purpose of such co-ordination is obvious; but again the mechanism is not known.

There are many other examples of integration leading to synchronous activity in all parts of the body, such as the hardening and darkening of the cuticle, the secretion of the waterproofing waxes, and, indeed, all the successive steps in the complex process of moulting and cuticle formation. It seems unlikely that each of these acts should be set going by some specific hormone. When the few proved hormonal stimuli have been considered, we are left with a large unexplained residue of integrated activities. Can we formulate any general hypothesis which would account for these in physiological terms?

In discussing the determination of bristles and plaques in the integument, it was suggested that a developing plaque absorbs some essential component from the region of the epidermis around it, so that determination of new plaques in the vicinity of an existing plaque is inhibited. Now it is possible to express this idea in more general terms and to say that the presence of two neighboring bristle-forming centres alters the chemical environment of the intervening epidermal cells in such a way that none of them becomes differentiated.

We extended this idea to describe the successive differentiations in a uniform tissue which is characteristic of the formation of all organs (p. 111). It is possible to extend the idea still further and to think of the circulating body fluid as a medium whose chemical properties will be influenced by the activities of all the various tissues that it bathes. Thus a sensitive mechanism for the detection of such activities by distant tissues would be provided.

The argument that we have been developing in this chapter is that the well-recognized means of integration from a distance, nervous conduction and hormone secretion, are merely specializations of properties that exist in generalized form in the epidermis.

The further suggestion that is being made now is that beyond the well-defined hormones, the products of the glands of internal secretion, there is a continual passage of chemical products to and from the various organs and tissues which could convey information from one part of the body to another.

The mammalian physiologist has long been familiar with the quasi-hormonal role of carbon dioxide or lactic acid as stimulators of the respiratory centre, with the products of fatigued muscles which inhibit voluntary effort and protect these muscles from overexertion, and with the effect of a fall in the blood-sugar level on the mobilization of carbohydrates.

To generalize these conceptions in order to provide a physiological mechanism for the integration of growth is to put forward a hypothesis that could be useful not only as a background for thought but as a basis for experiment.

Since the days of the Greek philosophers, it has been common practice to compare the integration of the body with the co-ordination of society. It is instructive to make such a comparison between the body of the insect and the communities of social Hymenoptera.

These insects have a highly developed central nervous system with elaborate organs of sensory perception; and there are plenty of examples of co-ordination among them that are dependent on specific acts of sensory communication. But over and above these reactions, there seems to be a response on the part of its individual members, either in behaviour or in morphogenetic development, to the needs of the society as a whole. There is much evidence, in ants and in the honeybee, that the mechanism for the communication of this information is "food sharing."

In the honeybee, every load of food that is brought into the hive is rapidly shared throughout the whole community. Ribbands and his colleagues[61] took six foraging bees from a colony of some 25,000 and allowed them to collect 20 ml. of sugar syrup containing $100\mu C$ of phosphorus–32. Two hours later 62 per cent of the forager bees and 19 per cent of all bees in the hive were radioactive. Within twenty-four hours 60 per cent of the bees had taken up internally the radioactive phosphorus.

Here is a mechanism by which every individual may be kept informed, from moment to moment, of the state and of the needs of the whole society. All can know whether the queen is still present and producing her characteristic secretion, whether water is in adequate supply, or whether there is a shortage of protein brought in by the pollen collectors. A resulting change in behaviour may serve to meet these needs; or the activation of appropriate genes by the changed nutrition of the brood may lead to alterations in the relative numbers of the different castes.

I suggest that we should apply this conception to the living animal. We should think of the tissue fluids as the vehicle for "food sharing" in the body—a vehicle for chemical communication which can lead to the integration of the growing organism in a way that finds a striking parallel in the integration of the communities of social insects.*

* In a more elaborate model on similar lines suggested by Weiss and Kavanau[80] the catalytic actions of certain key compounds ("templates") are pictured as being responsible for the reproduction of the specific

We spoke earlier of the essential organism being a chemical continuum, a giant molecule. Now we are speaking of it as a discontinuous community linked by a nexus of chemical exchanges. There is no contradiction here: the one system differentiates into the other; and this in turn develops into an organism with still more specialized modes of integration, well-defined hormones and nerves. The picture at which we arrive is a hypothetical one. But it is a reasonable one; for it represents the living organism as a hierarchy of integrative mechanisms rising from those of simple chemistry to those of the most complex physiology, with no break in the chain.

---

cytoplasm of each cell type. Each cell is also pictured as producing diffusible compounds antagonistic to these templates ("antitemplates"). According to this conception growth regulation occurs automatically by a negative "feedback" in which increasing numbers of antitemplates progressively block the corresponding templates.

References

1. AGRELL, I. (1952). The aerobic and anaerobic utilization of metabolic energy during insect metamorphosis. *Acta Physiol. Scand.* 28: 306–335.

2. ALLEN, T. H. (1940). Cytochrome oxidase in relation to respiratory activity and growth of the grasshopper egg. *J. Cell. Comp. Physiol.* 16: 149–163.

3. ASTAUROFF, B. L. (1930). Analyse der erblichen Störungsfälle der bilateralen Symmetrie im Zusammenhang mit der selbständigen Variabilität ähnlicher Strukturen. *Z. Indukt. Abstamm.–u. VererbLehre* 55: 183–262.

4. BEAMENT, J. W. L. (1945). The cuticular lipoids of insects. *J. Exp. Biol.* 21: 483–534.

5. BEAMENT, J. W. L. (1959). The waterproofing mechanism of arthropods. 1. The effect of temperature on cuticular permeability in terrestrial insects and ticks. *J. Exp. Biol.* 36: 391–422.

6. BODENSTEIN, D. (1953). Studies on the humoral mechanisms in growth and metamorphosis of the cockroach, *Periplaneta americana*. I. Transplantations of integumental structures and experimental parabioses. *J. Exp. Zool.* 123: 189–232.

REFERENCES

7. BODINE, J. H., and BOELL, E. J. (1934). Respiratory mechanisms of normally developing and blocked embryonic cells (Orthoptera). *J. Cell. Comp. Physiol.* 5: 97–113.

8. BOUNHIOL, J. J. (1938). Recherches expérimentales sur le déterminisme de la métamorphose chez les Lépidoptères. *Bull. biol. Suppl.* 24: 1–199.

9. BRIDGES, C. B., and DOBZHANSKY, T. (1933). The mutant "proboscipedia" in *Drosophila melanogaster*—a case of hereditary homoösis. *Roux Arch. EntwMech. Organ.* 127: 575–590.

10. BROWN, C. H. (1950). A review of the methods available for the determination of the types of forces stabilizing structural proteins in animals. *Quart. J. Micr. Sci.* 91: 331–339.

11. BURTT, E. T. (1938). On the corpora allata of dipterous insects II. *Proc. Roy. Soc.* B, 126: 210–223.

12. BUTENANDT, A., and KARLSON, P. (1954). Über die Isolierung eines Metamorphose–Hormones der Insekten in kristallisierter Form. *Z. Naturf.* 9b: 389–391.

13. BUTENANDT, A., KARLSON, P., and HANNES, G. (1946). Über den "Anti-bar-stoff," einen genabhängigen, morphogenetischen Wirkstoff bei *Drosophila melanogaster*. *Biol. Zbl.* 65:41–51.

14. BUXTON, P. A. (1930). The biology of the blood-sucking bug, *Rhodnius prolixus*. *Trans. R. Ent. Soc. Lond.* 78: 227–234.

15. CHEVAIS, S. (1943). Déterminisme de la taille de l'œil chez le mutant *Bar* de la Drosophile: intervention d'une substance diffusible spécifique. *Bull. biol.* 77: 1–108.

16. CHILD, C. M. (1941). *Patterns and problems of development*. Chicago: University of Chicago Press. 811 pp.

REFERENCES

17. CHURCH, N. S. (1955). Hormones and the termination and reinduction of diapause in *Cephus cinctus* Nort. (Hymenoptera: Cephidae). *Canad. J. Zool.* 33: 339–369.

18. DANIELLI, J. F. (1958). Studies of inheritance in amoebae by the technique of nuclear transfer. *Proc. Roy. Soc. Lond.* B, 148: 321–331.

19. EPHRUSSI, B. (1942). Chemistry of "eye colour hormones" of *Drosophila. Quart. Rev. Biol.* 17:326–338.

20. FORD, E. B. (1945). Polymorphism. *Biol. Rev.* 20: 73–88.

21. FRAENKEL, G. (1935). A hormone causing pupation in the blowfly *Calliphora erythrocephala. Proc. Roy. Soc.* B, 118: 1–12.

22. FUKUDA, S. (1940). Hormonal control of moulting and pupation in the silkworm. *Proc. Imp. Acad. Japan.* 16: 417–420.

23. FUKUDA, S. (1944). The hormonal mechanism of larval moulting and metamorphosis in the silkworm. *J. Fac. Sci. Tokyo Univ.* sec. IV, 6: 477–532.

24. GILBERT, L. I., and SCHNEIDERMAN, H. A. (1958). Occurrence of substances with juvenile hormone activity in adrenal cortex of vertebrates. *Science* 128: 844.

25. GLOOR, H. (1947). Phänokopie-Versuche mit Äther an *Drosophila. Rev. suisse zool.* 54: 637–712.

26. GOLDSCHMIDT, R. (1927). *Physiologische Theorie der Vererbung.* Berlin: Springer.

27. GOLDSCHMIDT, R. (1931). Analysis of intersexuality in the gipsy-moth. *Quart. Rev. Biol.* 6: 125–142.

28. GORDON, C., and SANG, J. H. (1941). The relation between nutrition and exhibition of the gene Antennaless *(Drosophila melanogaster). Proc. Roy. Soc.* B, 130: 151–184.

REFERENCES

29. HACHLOW, V. (1931). Zur Entwicklungsmechanik der Schmetterlinge. *Roux Arch. EntwMech. Organ.* 125: 26–49.

30. HACKMAN, R. H., and GOLDBERG, M. (1958). Proteins of the larval cuticle of *Agrianome spinicollis* (Coleoptera). *J. Ins. Physiol.* 2: 221–231.

31. HADORN, E. (1948). Genetische und entwicklungsphysiologische Probleme der Insektenontogenese. *Folia biotheor., Leiden* no. 3, pp. 109–126.

32. HADORN, E., and NEEL, J. (1938). Der hormonale Einfluss der Ringdrüse (corpus allatum) auf die Pupariumbildung bei Fliegen. *Roux Arch. EntwMech. Organ.* 138: 281–304.

33. HANSTRÖM, B. (1938). Zwei Probleme betreffs der hormonalen Lokalisation im Insektenkopf. *Acta Univ. Lund.* N.F., Avd. 2, 39: 1–17.

34. HANSTRÖM, B. (1940). Inkretorische Organe, Sinnesorgane und Nervensystem des Kopfes einiger niederer Insektenordnungen. *K. Svenska VetensAkad. Handl.* 18: 3–265.

35. HANSTRÖM, B. (1953). Neurosecretory pathways in the head of crustaceans, insects, and vertebrates. *Nature, Lond.* 171: 72–73.

36. HOLTFRETER, J. (1948). Concepts on the mechanism of embryonic induction and its relation to parthenogenesis and malignancy. *Symp. Soc. Exp. Biol.* 2: 17–49.

37. KENNEDY, J. S. (1956). Phase transformation in locust biology. *Biol. Rev.* 31: 349–370.

38. KLOOT, W. G. VAN DER (1955). The control of neurosecretion and diapause by physiological changes in the brain of the Cecropia silkworm. *Biol. Bull., Woods Hole* 109: 276–294.

REFERENCES

39. KOBAYASHI, M., and KIRIMURA, J. (1958). The "brain" hormone in the silkworm, *Bombyx mori* L. *Nature* 181: 1217.

40. KOPEČ, S. (1917). Experiments on metamorphosis of insects. *Bull. int. acad. Cracovie* B, pp. 57–60.

41. KOPEČ, S. (1922). Studies on the necessity of the brain for the inception of insect metamorphosis. *Biol. Bull., Woods Hole* 42: 322–342.

42. LOCKE, M. (1959). *J. Exp. Biol.* (in the press).

43. LOEB, J. (1913). *Artificial Parthenogenesis and Fertilization.* Chicago: University of Chicago Press.

44. LUBBOCK, J. (1883). *The Origin and Metamorphosis of Insects.* London: Macmillan.

45. LÜSCHER, M. (1958). Experimentelle Erzeugung von Soldaten bei der Termite *Kalotermes flavicollis* (Fabr.). *Naturwissenschaften* 45: 69–70.

46. MAAS, A. H. (1948). Über die Auslösbarkeit von Temperaturmodifikationen während der Embryonal-Entwicklung von *Drosophila melanogaster* Meigen. *Roux Arch. EntwMech. Organ.* 143: 515–572.

47. MOSCONA, A. (1957). The development *in vitro* of chimeric aggregates of dissociated embryonic chick and mouse cells. *Proc. Nat. Acad. Sci.* 43: 184–194.

48. NAYAR, K. K. (1954). Metamorphosis in the integument of caterpillars with omission of the pupal stage. *Proc. R. Ent. Soc. Lond.* A, 29: 129–134.

49. NOVAK, V. J. A. (1951). New aspects of the metamorphosis of insects. *Nature, Lond.* 167: 132–133.

50. O'FARRELL, A. F., and STOCK, A. (1953). Regeneration and the moulting cycle in *Blattella germanica* L. *Australian J. Biol. Sci.* 6:485–500.

REFERENCES

51. Passonneau, J. V., and Williams, C. M. (1953). The moulting fluid of the Cecropia silkworm. *J. Exp. Biol.* 30: 545–560.

52. Pflugfelder, O. (1937). Bau, Entwicklung und Funktion der Corpora allata und cardiaca von *Dixippus morosus* Br. *Z. wiss. Zool.* A, 149: 477–512.

53. Piepho, H. (1939a). Raupenhäutungen bereits verpuppter Hautstücke bei der Wachsmotte *Galleria mellonella* L. *Naturwissenschaften* 27: 301–302.

54. Piepho, H. (1939b). Über den Determinationszustand der Vorpuppenhypodermis bei der Wachsmotte *Galleria mellonella* L. *Biol. Zbl.* 59: 314–326.

55. Piepho, H. (1955). Über die polare Orientierung der Bälge und Schuppen auf den Schmetterlingsrumpf. *Biol. Zbl.* 74: 467–474.

56. Piepho, H., and Marcus, W. (1957). Wirkungen richtender Faktoren bei der Bildung der Schuppen und Bälge des Schmetterlingsrumpfes. *Biol. Zbl.* 76: 23–27.

57. Piepho, H., and Meyer, H. (1951). Reaktionen der Schmetterlingshaut auf Häutungshormone. *Biol. Zbl.* 70: 252–260.

58. Possompès, B. (1953). Recherches expérimentales sur le déterminisme de la métamorphose de *Calliphora erythrocephala* Meig. *Arch. zool. exp. gén.* 89: 203–364.

59. Pryor, M. G. M. (1940). On the hardening of the cuticle of insects. *Proc. Roy. Soc.* B, 128: 393–407.

60. Rahm, U. H. (1952). Die innersekretorische Steuerung der postembryonalen Entwicklung von *Sialis lutaria* L. (Megaloptera). *Rev. suisse zool.* 59: 173–237.

61. Ribbands, C. R., Kalmus, H., and Nixon, H. L. (1952). New evidence of communication in the honey bee colony. *Nature* 170: 438–440.

REFERENCES

62. RUNNSTRÖM, J. (1928). Struktur und Atmung bei der Entwicklungserregung des Seeigeleies. *Acta Zool.* 9: 445–499.

63. RUNNSTRÖM, J. (1949). *Advanc. Enzymol.* 9: 241–270.

64. SALT, G. (1927). The effects of stylopization on aculeate Hymenoptera. *J. Exp. Zool.* 48: 223–331.

65. SALT, G. (1931). A further study of the effects of stylopization on wasps. *J. Exp. Zool.* 59: 133–166.

66. SALT, G. (1937). The egg-parasite of *Sialis lutaria:* a study of the influence of the host upon a dimorphic parasite. *Parasitology* 29: 539–553.

67. SALT, G. (1938). Further notes on *Trichogramma semblidis. Parasitology* 30: 511–522.

68. SALT, G. (1941). The effects of hosts upon their insect parasites. *Biol. Rev.* 16: 239–264.

69. SALT, G. (1952). Trimorphism in the ichneumonid parasite *Gelis. Quart. J. Micr. Sci.* 93: 453–474.

70. SCHALLER, F. (1952). Effets d'une ligature postcéphalique sur le développement de larves agées d' *Apis mellifica* L. *Bull. soc. zool. Fr.* 77: 195–204.

71. SCHARRER, B. (1952). Neurosecretion. XI. The effects of nerve section on the intercerebralis-cardiacum-allatum system of the insect *Leucophaea maderae. Biol. Bull., Woods Hole* 102: 261–272.

72. SCHMIEDER, R. G. (1939). The significance of the two types of larvae in *Sphecophaga burra* (Cresson) and the factors conditioning them (Hym: Ichneumonidae). *Ent. News,* 50: 125–131.

73. SHAPPIRIO, D. C., and WILLIAMS, C. M. (1957). The cytochrome system of the Cecropia silkworm. *Proc. Roy. Soc. Lond.* B, 147: 218–246.

REFERENCES

74. THOMSEN, E. (1942). An experimental and anatomical
study of the corpus allatum in the blow-fly *Calliphora
erythrocephala* Meig. *Vidensk. Medd. dansk. naturh.
Foren. Kbh.* 106: 319–405.

75. THOMSEN, E., and MØLLER, I. (1959). *Nature,* 183:
1401–1402.

76. VILLEE, C. A. (1943). Phenogenetic studies of the homo-
eotic mutants of *Drosophila melanogaster.* (i) The effects
of temperature on the expression of aristopedia. *J. Exp.
Zool.* 93: 75–98.

77. VILLEE, C. A. (1944). Phenogenetic studies of the homo-
eotic mutants of *Drosophila melanogaster.* (ii) The effects
of temperature on the expression of proboscipedia. *J.
Exp. Zool.* 96: 85–102.

78. VOGT, M. (1943). Zur Produktion und Bedeutung meta-
morphosefördernder Hormone während der Larvenent-
wicklung von *Drosophila.* *Biol. Zbl.* 63: 395–446.

79. WEBER, R. (1958). Über die submikroskopische Organi-
sation und die biochemische Kennzeichnung embryonaler
Entwicklungsstadien von *Tubifex.* *Roux Arch. Entw-
Mech. Organ.* 150: 542–580.

80. WEISS, P., and KAVANAU, J. L. (1957). A model of
growth and growth control in mathematical terms. *J.
Gen. Physiol.* 41: 1–47.

81. WELLS, M. J., and WELLS, J. (1959). Hormonal control
of sexual maturity in *Octopus.* *J. Exp. Biol.* 36: 1–33.

82. WIEDBRAUCK, H. (1953). Wiederholung der Metamorphose von Schmetterlingshaut. Versuche an der Wachsmotte *Galleria mellonella* L. *Biol. Zbl.* 72: 530–562.

83. WIGGLESWORTH, V. B. (1933). The physiology of the
cuticle and of ecdysis in *Rhodnius prolixus* (Triatomidae,
Hemiptera); with special reference to the function of the

oenocytes and of the dermal glands. *Quart. J. Micr. Sci.* 76: 269–318.

84. WIGGLESWORTH, V. B. (1934). The physiology of ecdysis in *Rhodnius prolixus* (Hemiptera). II. Factors controlling moulting and "metamorphosis." *Quart. J. Micr. Sci.* 77: 191–222.

85. WIGGLESWORTH, V. B. (1936). The function of the corpus allatum in the growth and reproduction of *Rhodnius prolixus* (Hemiptera). *Quart. J. Micr. Sci.* 79: 91–121.

86. WIGGLESWORTH, V. B. (1937). Wound healing in an insect *(Rhodnius prolixus* Hemiptera). *J. Exp. Biol.* 14: 364–381.

87. WIGGLESWORTH, V. B. (1939). Häutung bei Imagines von Wanzen. *Naturwissenschaften* 27: 301.

88. WIGGLESWORTH, V. B. (1940*a*). Local and general factors in the development of "pattern" in *Rhodnius prolixus* (Hemiptera). *J. Exp. Biol.* 17: 180–200.

89. WIGGLESWORTH, V. B. (1940*b*). The determination of characters at metamorphosis in *Rhodnius prolixus* (Hemiptera). *J. Exp. Biol.* 17: 201–222.

90. WIGGLESWORTH, V. B. (1942). The significance of "chromatic droplets" in the growth of insects. *Quart. J. Micr. Sci.* 83: 141–152.

91. WIGGLESWORTH, V. B. (1945*a*). Transpiration through the cuticle of insects. *J. Exp. Biol.* 21: 97–114.

92. WIGGLESWORTH, V. B. (1945*b*). Growth and form in an insect. *Essays on Growth and Form.* Oxford: Oxford University Press.

93. WIGGLESWORTH, V. B. (1947). The epicuticle in an insect *Rhodnius prolixus* (Hemiptera). *Proc. Roy. Soc.* B, 134: 163–181.

REFERENCES

94. WIGGLESWORTH, V. B. (1948a). The functions of the corpus allatum in *Rhodnius prolixus* (Hemiptera). *J. Exp. Biol.* 25: 1–14.

95. WIGGLESWORTH, V. B. (1948b). The structure and deposition of the cuticle in the adult mealworm, *Tenebrio molitor* L. (Coleoptera). *Quart. J. Micr. Sci.* 89: 197–217.

96. WIGGLESWORTH, V. B. (1948c). The role of the cell in determination. *Symp. Soc. Exp. Biol.* 2: 1–16.

97. WIGGLESWORTH, V. B. (1948d). The insect cuticle. *Biol. Rev.* 23: 408–451.

98. WIGGLESWORTH, V. B. (1949). The utilization of reserve substances in *Drosophila* during flight. *J. Exp. Biol.* 26: 150–163.

99. WIGGLESWORTH, V. B. (1952a). The thoracic gland in *Rhodnius prolixus* (Hemiptera) and its role in moulting. *J. Exp. Biol.* 29: 561–570.

100. WIGGLESWORTH, V. B. (1952b). Hormone balance and the control of metamorphosis in *Rhodnius prolixus* (Hemiptera). *J. Exp. Biol.* 29: 620–631.

101. WIGGLESWORTH, V. B. (1953). The origin of sensory neurones in an insect, *Rhodnius prolixus* (Hemiptera). *Quart. J. Micr. Sci.* 94: 93–112.

102. WIGGLESWORTH, V. B. (1954a). Secretion of juvenile hormone by the corpus allatum of *Calliphora*. *Nature* 174: 556.

103. WIGGLESWORTH, V. B. (1954b). *The physiology of insect metamorphosis*. Cambridge: Cambridge University Press. 152 pp.

104. WIGGLESWORTH, V. B. (1955a). The breakdown of the thoracic gland in the adult insect, *Rhodnius prolixus*. *J. Exp. Biol.* 32: 485–491.

105. WIGGLESWORTH, V. B. (1955*b*). The role of the haemocytes in the growth and moulting of an insect, *Rhodnius prolixus* (Hemiptera). *J. Exp. Biol.* 32: 649–663.

106. WIGGLESWORTH, V. B. (1956*a*). The haemocytes and connective tissue formation in an insect, *Rhodnius prolixus* (Hemiptera). *Quart. J. Micr. Sci.* 97: 89–98.

107. WIGGLESWORTH, V. B. (1956*b*). Formation and involution of striated muscle fibres during the growth and moulting cycles of *Rhodnius prolixus* (Hemiptera). *Quart. J. Micr. Sci.* 97: 465–480.

108. WIGGLESWORTH, V. B. (1957*a*). The physiology of insect cuticle. *Ann. Rev. Ent.* 2: 37–54.

109. WIGGLESWORTH, V. B. (1957*b*). The action of growth hormones in insects. *Symp. Soc. Exp. Biol.* 11: 204–227.

110. WIGGLESWORTH, V. B. (1958*a*). Abrasion of the insect cuticle by aqueous suspensions of small particles. *Nature* 181: 779–780.

111. WIGGLESWORTH, V. B. (1958*b*. Some methods for assaying extracts of the juvenile hormone in insects. *J. Ins. Physiol.* 2: 73–84.

112. WILLIAMS, C. M. (1947). Physiology of insect diapause. II. Interaction between the pupal brain and prothoracic glands in the metamorphosis of the giant silkworm, *Platysamia cecropia*. *Biol. Bull., Woods Hole* 93: 89–98.

113. WILLIAMS, C. M. (1951). Biochemical mechanisms in insect growth and metamorphosis. *Fed. Proc.* 10: 546–552.

114. WILLIAMS, C. M. (1952). Morphogenesis and the metamorphosis of insects. *Harvey Lectures* 47: 126–155.

115. WILLIAMS, C. M. (1956*a*). The juvenile hormone in insects. *Nature* 178: 212–213.

116. WILLIAMS, C. M. (1956*b*). Personal communication.

REFERENCES

117. WILLIAMS, C. M., MOORHEAD, L. V., and PULIS, J. F. (1959). Juvenile hormone in thymus, human placenta and other mammalian organs. *Nature* 183: 405.

118. WOLSKY, A. (1938). The effect of carbon monoxide on the oxygen consumption of *Drosophila melanogaster* pupae. *J. Exp. Biol.* 15: 225–234.

119. WOLSKY, A. (1941). Quantitative changes in the substrate-dehydrogenase system of *Drosophila* pupae during metamorphosis. *Science* 94: 48–49.

120. ZWICKY, K., and WIGGLESWORTH, V. B. (1956). The course of oxygen consumption during the moulting cycle of *Rhodnius prolixus* Stål (Hemiptera). *Proc. R. Ent. Soc. Lond.* A., 31: 153–160.

The Messenger Lectures

IN its original form this book consisted of six lectures delivered at Cornell University in October, 1958, namely, the Messenger Lectures on the Evolution of Civilization. That series was founded and its title prescribed by Hiram J. Messenger, B. Litt., Ph.D., of Hartford, Connecticut, who directed in his will that a portion of his estate be given to Cornell University and used to provide annually a "course or courses of lectures on the evolution of civilization, for the special purpose of raising the moral standard of our political, business, and social life." The lectureship was established in 1923.

Index

Acetabularia, 2
Acrasia, 3
Acrasin, 109
Activation, 51
Amoeba, 2, 5
Amphibia, 3
Autolysis, 107

Bacteria, 1
Basement membrane, 14
Burns, repair of, 71

Castes, 122
Castration, 43
Cell affinity, 37
Cell death, 105
Cement layer, 12
Chitin, 9
Cholinesterase, 48
Chromatin droplets, 105
Cleavage nuclei, 113
Competence, 92
Corpus allatum, 45, 76
Corpus cardiacum, 47
Critical period, 44, 75
Cuticle, 6
Cuticulin, 9
Cytochrome C, 63
Cytochrome system, 54
Cytoskeleton, 40

Dermal glands, 12
Determination of dermal glands, 29

Determination of sensilla, 26
Diapause, 54
Differentiation, 21

Ecdyson, 50
Echinoderms, 3
Embryonic development, 111
Embryos, 3
Endopterygota, 70
Epidermal cell, 6
Evocators, 98
Expression, 97

Fat body, 56
Field, 32
Food sharing, 122

Genetics, 3
Giant larvae, 77
Goldschmidt's theory, 80
Gonad development, 90
Gradient theory, 31, 112

Haemocytes, 14, 118
Hemimetabola, 67
Hibernation, 54
Histolysis, 106
Holometabola, 67
Hormones, 4

Imaginal discs, 70
Induction, 3
Inductors, 32, 99

INDEX

Inhibitory hormone, 80
Insects, 6
Integration of growth, 105
Intersexes, 99

Juvenile hormone, 87

Macronucleus, 112
Malignant growth, 4
Melanism, 96
Metamorphosis, 67
Metathetely, 92
Mimicry, 96
Mitochondria, 57
Modifier, 32
Moulting, 7
Moulting fluid, 11
Moulting hormone, 44
Muscles, 57
Mutant genes, 96

Neotenin, 87
Neoteny, 102
Nerve regeneration, 38
Neurilemma cell, 35
Neurosecretory cells, 45, 115
Nutrition and morphogenesis, 101

Oenocytes, 16, 22
Orientation of bristles, 40

Paramoecium, 1
Pattern, 74
Penetrance, 96
Phase change, 101
Planarians, 2
Polyeidism, 95
Polymorphism, 91
Pore canals, 9
Protein synthesis, 62
Proteolytic enzymes, 63
Prothetely, 91

Prothoracic gland, 45
Protozoa, 1, 112
Puberty, 90
Pupa, 92
Puparium, 44

Quinone tanning, 13

Regeneration, 4, 26, 119
Repair, 4
Respiration rate, 56
Reversal of metamorphosis, 88
Rhodnius, 5
Ring gland, 45

Sclerotin, 13
Sense cell, 19, 35
Sense organs, 18
Sensillum, 35
Sensory axon, 35
Sensory bristle, 22
Sex, 99
Slime mould, 3
Social insects, 121
Sponges, 3
Superadult, 102
Superlarva, 102
Synchronous activity, 120

Termites, 102
Thoracic glands, 46, 106
Tormogen cell, 35
Trichogen cell, 35
Tyrosinase, 12

Viruses, 1

Wax, 11
Wound healing, 37, 108

Yolk formation, 77